BUILDING HEALTHY LUNGS "NATURALLY"

First © January 2004 by Michael Grant White, LMBT • NE • OBDMT
Revised © January 2005

Edited by: Jan Jenson, Earnestine Nix and Kay Graybeal
Layout by: Jan Jenson • The WELLth Coach!

Copyright
No part of this book may be reproduced or utilized in any form or by any means, electronic or mechanical, including photocopying, recording, or by any information storage and retrieval system without written permission from Michael Grant White at: www.breathing.com/contact.htm or by calling 1-866-694-6425 or 866 My Inhale

Medical Disclaimer:
Exercises or advice given in this book are not intended to replace the services of your physician, or to provide an alternative to professional medical treatment. This book offers no diagnosis or treatment for any specific medical problem. When we suggest the possible usefulness of certain practices in relation to certain illnesses or symptoms, it is for educational purposes — either to explore the relationship of natural breathing to health or to expose the reader to alternative healing approaches. **At the first suspicion of any disease or disorder please consult a licensed primary health care professional. Bring this book with you.** Second and third opinions are often quite valuable especially when drugs and/or surgery are involved. Make sure your health professional knows about our Optimal Breathing® Development System before they administer their services. Unless you have no other practical choice, don't just "go with" what you're told first!" — Michael Grant White

All rights reserved. Permission to quote up to 100 words gladly given by crediting **Building Healthy Lungs, Naturally: Biochemical and Environmental Aspects of the Optimal Breathing Development System**, "Michael Grant White, Breathing Development Specialist' and a copy of the publication sent to address on Breathing.com website. Written permission required for larger passages. Otherwise, no part of this writing may be copied or reproduced or utilized in any form or by any means, electronic or mechanical, including photocopying, recording, or by any information storage and retrieval system without written permission from the author.

Goals and purposes of Optimal Breathing®

- To show traditional and alternative health professionals and associated professions exactly HOW to utlize the fundamentals of Optimal Breathing®, and in doing so;
- To enhance their services with ours and apply their newly integrated/holistic paradigm for all patients, clients, teachers and students' unique needs.
- To give new hope to the sick and dying.
- To give internal power and energy to people in need.
- To attract and educate people who want to take responsibility for their health and longevity.
- To help people realize that all non-surgically altered and congenitally normal humans breathe the same way and that everyone can learn to breathe better.
- To bring awareness to simple approaches and practices everyone best for them for their unique health, performance and life extension.
- To help people to realize the emerging patterns, rising out of our primitive and enduring "suck, swallow, breathe" reflexes.
- To motivating everyone to reflect on the extent to which these patterns greatly influence who we are and what we do as we unfold our lives one breath at a time.
- To help people realize that the way they breathe CAN be incredibly inspirational, and that it is their intention that makes it so, resulting in their improved breathing becoming a major priority. They can inturn inspire others to learn about Optimal Breathing® Development.
- To restore and strengthen our faith in who we are and who we want to be.

With Optimal Breathing® as our foundation, we have a lot more to say about our present and future than we ever thought possible.

BUILDING HEALTHY LUNGS "NATURALLY"

Table of Contents
INTRODUCTION   9

CHAPTERS
1. Mechanical Breathing Function   22
2. Posture & Ergonomics   27
3. Movement and lung function   34
4. Breathing Exercises   38
5. Squeeze and breathe   42
6. Diet & Nutrition   45
7. Digestion and elimination - just as important as healthy eating   66
8. Sunshine   73
9. Water   77
10. Supplements - including 55 lung-friendly ones   82
11. Hair, Urine & Blood Testing- $ave a lot of money   93
12. Fasting, cleansing   95
13. Detoxification – food, air, environment, cosmetics   109
14. Weight control   136
15. Lung Diseases   141
16. 300 meds that can harm the lungs   149
17. Oxygen therapies   152
18. Testimonials touch all who are living because "Breath is Life"   154

Results from over 40,000 free breathing tests at http://www.breathing.com/test.htm have convinced me that poor breathing is connected with virtually every illness or compromised human ability. Breath is life. But the big questions are WHY, HOW and WHEN is breath life?

APPENDIX   173
Recommended Websites   173
Recommended Books   175
Websites for Courses to take, products, recipes   177

OPTIMAL BREATHING SCHOOL   179

** ORDER OPTIMAL BREATHING® PRODUCTS**   184
Books; DVDs/Videos; CD/cassettes; Nutritional products

Do you know that Optimal Breathing® does not come naturally?
It is a **LEARNED SKILL**.
We ALL need to breathe optimally
and we ALL can learn to breathe at a much more optimal level.

BUILDING HEALTHY LUNGS "NATURALLY"

Biochemical and Environmental Aspects of the Optimal Breathing Development System

Companion book to:
- ✘ Secrets of Optimal Breathing® Development (Manual)
- ✘ Fundamentals of Optimal Breathing Development DVD #176
- ✘ The Way You Breathe Can Make You Sick or Make You Well
- ✘ Sleeping, Snoring & the Stress Level Elimination Energy Plan — S.L.E.E.P.

The Optimal Breathing® System is comprised of:

A. Secrets of Optimal Breathing Manual – A synthesis of 30 years of research related to the authors' personal quest to regain healthy breathing. It addresses the vast range of supplemental breathing development techniques learned from my 30 years experience and includes insights from more than 40,000 online test results from my website: http://www.breathing.com/tests.htm. This enhances self teaching and enables me and the Optimal Breathing School staff and graduates to help others with singing, athletics, meditating, laughing, bliss, crying, speaking out, performing delicate tasks, and recovering from stress of habitual activities that cause shallow or distorted breathing

B. The Fundamentals Of Optimal Breathing Development DVD #176. Benefits include: A great deal of chest expansion and increased volume and ease of breathing. Exercises and strapping techniques demonstrated on the DVD/video quickly and gently release tensions in the muscles of the rib cage to improve breathing ease, chest and lung shape and volume. These techniques help you use more of your vital capacity; ease heart function by freeing up the space the heart needs to expand in, and release unnecessary tension that keeps your breathing in an inefficient pattern. The exercises help you restore natural breathing rhythm while enhancing breathing sequencing and balance; reduce residual lung volume; reduction or elimination of excessively fast (rapid and/or hyperventilation) breathing; postural and breathing musculo-skeletal balancing; respiratory chemistry improvement; improves being in "present time", and ways of objectively marking progress. You will notice improvement immediately! This helps many troublesome or difficult/chronic health problems and often reduces or eliminates low back pain. Our techniques are compatible with all forms of exercise, performance, movement and therapy.

C. Building Healthy Lungs Naturally. This portion of our Optimal Breathing System is about key aspects of biochemical, toxicity and everything else EXCEPT the mechanical aspect of breathing development.

D. The Way You Breathe Can Make You Sick or Make You Well is a wake up call to alert you and offers ways of assessing if something is wrong with your breathing. Did you know the way you breathe can cause or worsen addictions, allergies, anxiety, asthma, bad memory, cancer, chest pains, depression, fatigue, forgetting to breathe, holding breath, low sex drive, overweight, panic attacks, phobias, poor voice quality, shortness of breath, being almost constantly stressed out trouble sleeping?

E. Sleeping, Snoring and the Stress Level Elimination Energy Plan (S.L.E.E.P.) addresses key aspects of our Optimal Healthy Stress Elimination Exercise Plan.

F. The Optimal Breathing School. A worldwide training and certification program in proprietary touch & non touch methods to rapidly develop natural breathing in your self, clients, patients, friends and loved ones without inflicting pain, drugs or surgery. The primary purpose of our school is to train leading edge traditional and alternative modality practitioners, plus people interested in breathing development as a support for themselves, friends or loved ones. Because breath is life, our primary goal is to create a community of people and practitioners who breathe optimally. Our students and practitioners will carry forward the teaching of Optimal Breathing®.

G. The Optimal Breathing Development system is augmented by CDs/cassettes:

Recorded breathing exercises for:
1. Deeper Relaxation and Calming
2. Extra Energy
3. Mental Focus.
4. Self Esteem

Seminars, talk shows and workshops
1. Optimal Breathing Seminar at the 2001 Portland Raw foods Festival
2. The Breath of Life - a radio talk show discussing 15 things you must know about breathing to live a good life.

H. In addition we offer various products such as for nutrition and diet, homeopathics, protecting your respiration, mechanical breathing development aids, manuals, books and booklets here: http://www.breathing.com/programs.htm

I. The Breathing.com Web site has over 1,000 pages and 300 articles on a wide range of breathing related subjects.
http://www.breathing.com/articlesDefault.htm
PLUS a free weekly newsletter. http://www.breathing.com/subscribe.htm

Due to its immense size and the scope required by the subject of breathing, we encourage you to call or email if you have a question about your specific needs. FIRST take our free breathing tests so you have a better idea how we are trying to help you. http://www.breathing.com/tests.htm

BARRING HARMFUL ACCIDENTS, BIRTH DEFECTS AND CERTAIN SURGERIES, PRACTICALLY EVERY HEALTH GOAL CAN BE ATTAINED BY UTILIZING A HOLISTIC COMBINATION OF:
- **Cleansing & Fasting**
- **Detoxification Including Identifying Toxins In Personal Care & Cleaning Products, Air, Water, Foods, Environment**
- **Organic Live Nutrition**
- **Supplements**
- **Digestion & Elimination**
- **Prayer & Meditation**
- **Positive Affirmations**
- **Ergonomics**
- **Movement & Exercise**
- **Oxygen Therapies**

Do you know that Optimal Breathing does not come naturally?
It is a SKILL.
We ALL need to breathe and we ALL can learn to breathe much better!

ABOUT BREATHING

The mechanistic approach of modern science and the abstract and jargon-laden nature of spiritual and psychological explorations have obscured the mysteries and power of the breath. Why and how we breathe needs to be clarified for a simpler, common sense understanding.

Breathing involves the physical and mechanical acts of muscles, chemicals, and neural activity that draw air into your body through expansion, contraction and pulsation. Structural, postural, muscular, energetic and hormonal aspects of your body support or inhibit this process.

Breath is the air or life force that is taken in. The influence your life force has on your breathing can alter, to a great degree, all aspects of your thought, experience and expression of life. As you grow from infancy to adulthood, your breath ebbs and flows and your body becomes an outward expression of your breathing freedom or restriction.

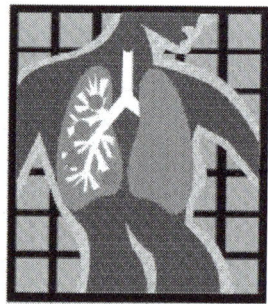

This portion of our Optimal Breathing® Develop-ment System (BHLN) addresses the biochemical and environmental aspects of breathing (mechanics) and respiration (chemistry).

"Breathing is the FIRST place not the LAST place one should investigate when any disordered energy presents itself."
— Sheldon Saul Hendler, MD Ph.D.

INTRODUCTION

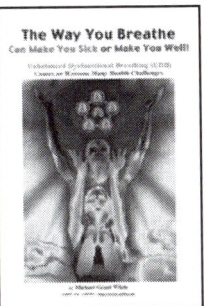

First, learn why you need to improve your breathing in *The Way You Breathe Can Make You Sick or Make You Well.* http://www.breathing.com/theway/htm   Then, if you have an interest, you can take our self-help courses and/or advanced training and become certified to teach others how to improve their breathing. Breathing is generic to all humanity, therefore all health care professionals will find breathing development a valuable addition to the services they offer.

You should invest in our most popular home study training programs:
Introductory: #176 DVD or video
http://www.breathing.com/176.htm
Advanced: Our Most Popular Program #250
http://www.breathing.com/250.htm
(The #250 program contains the #176 DVD/video and a LOT more valuable and useful information!)

Check our calendar of events for the days and place of the next scheduled **Optimal Breathing School**: http://www.breathing.com/school.htm

EVERYONE can greatly improve their breathing! But why bother learning about breathing at all?

THE PROMISE
"I believe that barring harmful accidents, birth defects and certain surgeries, practically every health goal CAN be attained with a holistic combination of breathing development, cleansing, fasting, organic live nutrition, vitamin/mineral supplements, prayer and meditation, positive daily affirmations, pure water, clean air and living environment, optimal ergonomics and moderate exercise.

Breathing properly allows us to run the full range of emotions, and yet come back to deep peace, etc. We become able, like the animals in the wild, to shake off our stress, become calm and recover in the shortest possible times. "Reasonable" is defined by our individual values. Hopefully we seek those values that support our highest way of being. If this is not achieved then it is not optimal. States of peace, love and joy are what my research leads me to believe is the physical body's natural state of being. It allows for the longest and most satisfying life." —
Michael Grant White

WHY SHOULD YOU DEVELOP YOUR BREATHING?

LEADING CAUSES OF DEATH IN THE U.S. in 2002
Heart Disease: 696,947
Cancer: 557,271
Pneumonia: 65,681
Stroke: 162,672
58,866

Diabetes: 73,249
Influenza/

Alzheimer's disease:

Chronic lower respiratory diseases: 124,816
Nephritis, nephrotic syndrome, nephrosis: 40,974
Accidents (unintentional injuries): 106,742   Septicemia: 33,865
_{(Source: Deaths/Mortality: Final Data for 2002: http://www.cdc.gov/nchs/fastats/deaths.htm}
Number of deaths: 2,443,387
Death rate: 845.3 deaths per 100,000 population
Life expectancy: 77.3 years
These statistics don't include the lack of oxygen factors for the first three causes of death, which all have a HUGE issue related to breathing!

Your best source of oxygen is the way you breathe so, MAKE THE CHEMISTRY AND MECHANICS OF YOUR BREATHING YOUR FIRST PRIORITY!

Heart attacks, cancer, strokes, pneumonia, asthma, speech problems and almost every disease known to mankind is worsened or improved by how well you breathe; the quality of your respiration.

Within certain limitations (i.e. genetic or surgical abnormalities), time and age of the individual, lung tissue can be revitalized. We focus somewhat on emphysema here to show others that even it can be improved and to use it as a role model and source of inspiration. You can utilize more aspects of this holistic program to progress faster.

Optimal Natural Breathing (ONB) addresses a Utopian or non-Utopian world in the best way possible. It is a qualified and quantified look and feel that is reflective of the best that can be had in the moment. It stems from a strong foundation and allows for freedom and depth and range of maximal experience. It allows for singing, athletics, meditating, laughing, bliss, crying, speaking out, performing delicate tasks, recovering from stress, or habitual activities that cause shallow or distorted breathing, the quickest and most thorough healing of wounds, illnesses, physical as well as emotional and spiritual.

ONB allows us to run the full range of emotions, yet go back to deep peace. We become able, like the animals in the wild, to shake off our stress, become calm and recover in the shortest possible time. "Reasonable" is defined by our individual values. Hopefully, we seek those values that support our highest way of being. If this is not achieved then it is not optimal, because states of peace, love and joy are what my research has lead me to believe is the physical body's natural state of being — it allows for the longest and most satisfying life!

Germs, viruses and bacteria are anaerobic: they cannot survive in high concentrations of oxygen. Breathing properly greatly increases oxygen levels in the body, thus reducing disease!

DO YOU OFTEN CATCH YOURSELF NOT BREATHING?

Do you experience shallow, labored breathing; shortness of breath; a high chest; stuck, erratic or reverse breathing? Are you unable to catch your breath? Do you have blue-tinted lips or fingernails; trouble sleeping; more than 6-8 resting breaths per minute with 3-6 second pauses; heart beat irregularities; poor posture, mild to severe depression; tightness across your chest; excessive stress; asthma or COPD symptoms; constant fatigue; chronic pain; chest pains; anger; anxiety; hyperventilation?

THE LUNGS CAN BE REACTIVATED

"Curing emphysema is possible. The lungs that medical science thought impossible to reactivate can in fact be reactivated". — **Robert Nims, M.D.** Pulmonary Specialist.

Your lungs become less active and actually shrink in size if you do not use them properly or abuse them through smoking, bad air or devitalized food. If you want to live as long and as healthy as possible, you need to offset that "shrinkage" and weakness with specific breathing exercises, lung expansion and diaphragm-enlarging techniques, clean air, moderate exercise, proper digestion, internal cleansing, and healthy nutrition.

Lung tissue, just like brain and heart tissue, thought previously to be lost to sickness or non-use, can be reactivated. Sadly, there is still little recognition that lung cells are renewable cells as well. I believe ALL cells, if still alive, can, to a reasonable degree, be brought back to significant function. When you can no longer revitalize the lungs you can enlarge the rib cage and make more room for what lung tissue you do have to be moved-squeezed and expanded more, which displaces debris and aids gas exchange, volume and ease of breathing.

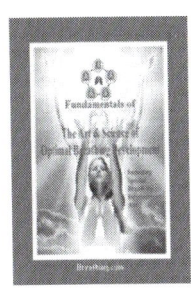

The exercises shown on our **#176 DVD** and using the **Diaphragm Strengthener** aid this expansion quite well.
http://www.breathing.com/video-ds.htm

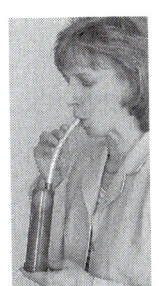

MOUNTING EVIDENCE FROM CLINICAL STUDIES

Clinical studies including thousands of participants spanning a 30-year period (Framingham Study) offer persuasive evidence that the most significant factor in health and longevity is how well you breathe.

The Framingham Study focused on the long-term predictive power of vital capacity and forced exhalation volume as the primary markers for life span. *"This pulmonary function measurement appears to be an indicator of general health and vigor and literally a measure of living capacity".* — **Wm B. Kannel and Helen Hubert.**

These researchers were able to foretell how long a person was going to live by measuring forced exhalation breathing volume, FEV1 and hypertension. We know that much of hypertension is controlled by the way we breathe. (Doing the exercises on our #176 DVD/video plus using the Diaphragm Strengthener will develop breathing volume.
http://www.breathing.com/video-ds.htm)

"Long before a person becomes terminally ill, vital capacity can predict life span." William B. Kannel of Boston School of Medicine (1981) stated, *"The Framingham exam's predictive powers were as accurate over the 30-year period as are more recent exams."* **The Study concluded that vital capacity falls 9 percent to 27 percent each decade depending on age, sex and the time the test is given.** The Study's shortcoming was in suggesting that vital capacity cannot be maintained and/or

increased, even in severe cases of chronic obstructive pulmonary disease (COPD).

Any opera (not necessarily voice) teacher will support the idea that breathing volume can be increased. Yet activities such as singing or sports are no guarantee of optimal breathing. In fact, they can even invite breathing blocks from gasping, forcing the exhale and breath heaving. You don't have to learn how to sing to have a huge pair of lungs. **But you DO need to know how to breathe properly.** I maintain that if you train someone to breathe correctly, they will naturally know how to sing. I've never seen it fail.

You can get the complete Framingham Study at the National Institute of Health's Database. http://www.ncbi.nlm.nih.gov/PubMed/ We provide copies of it for our Optimal Breathing School attendees. We also include magazine interviews with the leaders of the Study.

REMINDER: Most scientific research is and was done with rats and primates who do not breathe the same as humans. Researchers did not seem to believe (at that time) that you could improve your breathing. Many still do not believe anyone can improve their breathing. This is simply not true!

29 Years After The Framingham Study, The Same Conclusions Prevail.
Lung Function May Predict Long Life or Early Death

How well your lungs function may predict how long you live. This finding is the result of a nearly 30-year follow-up of the association between impaired pulmonary function and all causes of mortality. Researchers at the University at Buffalo conducted a study and their results appear in the September 2000 issue of *Chest*.

The purpose of the current study was to investigate the association between pulmonary function and mortality for periods that extended past 25 years, the limit of previous studies. Dr. Schunemann and colleagues also wanted to determine how and why poor pulmonary function is a significant predictor of mortality.

Results showed that lung function was a significant predictor of longevity in the whole group for the full 29 years of follow-up. *"It is important to note that the risk of death was increased for participants with moderately impaired lung function, not merely those in the lowest quintile,"* Dr. Schunemann said. *"This suggests that the increased risk isn't confined to a small fraction of the population with severely impaired lung function."*

"The reasons lung function may predict mortality are not clear," Dr. Schunemann said, noting that increased risk is found in persons who never smoked, as well as among smokers. *"The lung is a primary defense organism against environmental toxins. It could be that impaired pulmonary function could lead to decreased tolerance against these toxins. Researchers also have speculated that decreased pulmonary function could underlie an increase in oxidative stress from free radicals, and we know that oxidative stress plays a role in the development of many diseases."*

Dr. Schanemann said the fact that a relationship does exists between lung function and risk of death should motivate physicians to screen patients for pulmonary function, even if more research is needed to determine why. *"It is surprising that this simple measurement has not gained more importance as a general health assessment tool,"* **he noted.**

Schunemann HJ, Dorn J, Grant BJB, Winkelstein W, Jr., Trevisan M., *Pulmonary Function Is a Long-term Predictor of Mortality in the General Population 29-Year Follow-up of the Buffalo Health Study.* **Chest** 2000; 118(3) 656-664

From Mike: *"Surprising" is a masterpiece of understatement!" Decline in FEV1 (breathing volume) by age and smoking status: facts, figures and fallacies.* **Thorax** 1997 52:820-827.

This study shows the importance of longitudinal studies as opposed to cross sectional ones.

This published article focused on a compilation of 83 published reports and clinical studies showing clearly that the primary measurement for lung function -FEV1 - is based on cross sectional data instead of longitudinal data. This means essentially that they include sick people with widely diverse circumstances in their statistics and compile everyone's data for mass diagnosis.

This 1997 research paper points out that (italics Mike's) *"from one low measurement of FEV1 (forced exhalation volume) in an adult, it is impossible to determine whether the reduced lung function is due to not having achieved a high maximum during early adulthood, or to having an accelerated rate of decline or to any combination of these."* "Western medical studies, via cross sectioning, continue to look for role modeling epidemiological "norms" that include the ranks of the ill. Cross sectioning is 60% effective and proven by many to be ineffective over the last 40 years."

The health professional's opinion can have immense personal, social, legal, and economic consequences. When it is based on information colored by sick or otherwise non-optimum healthy or inappropriately chosen individuals, the statistic(s) become weighted in favor of, or excessively influenced by, illness or what is perceived as illness, and may well be in reality, simple mechanical dysfunction. Cross sectional studies can bring the averages down and cause many who do not need the intensity, duration or style of treatment recommended by many health practitioners to be over or under medicated, or inappropriately fed, exercised, massaged or educated.

Dwelling too much on problems and pathology (illness model) gets in the way of creativity and flexibility. We need to focus on how to improve breathing, not so much how it on how it became impaired. How is important so we do not repeat our mistakes but without the insights of the skills of optimal breathing development we will never know what direction to travel to attain the best possible breathing capabilities.

FAMOUS STUDENTS OF OXYGEN AND RESPIRATION

Dr. Manfred von Ardenne was a student of Dr. Otto Warburg, who received the 1931 Nobel Prize for proving that *cancer is anaerobic: it cannot survive in a high oxygen environment. Germs, fungi and bacteria are anaerobic as well.* von Ardenne was inspired by Karl Lohmann who discovered adenosine triphosphate (ATP), which many believe to be the human body's main energy currency. von Ardenne was an electron physicist, who in addition to his interest in astronomy, developed quite a good reputation for cancer research.

The von Ardenne studies focused on oxygen's relationship to most major categories of illness. *When your blood oxygen goes way down, you get sick, die or at least shorten your life span.* His book is a masterful compilation of clinical insights and variations on breathing assessments, co-factors and some techniques of breathing development he called **Oxygen Multi-step Therapy**. In his book of the same name, Dr. von Ardenne addressed at least 150 respiratory and blood gas aspects, including elements of what I call respiratory psychophysiology.

The von Ardenne material is good but remains primarily within the illness model instead of the wellness model.

Some studies addressed in von Ardenne's book include:
- Dependence of O_2 uptake at rest.
- The O_2 deficiency pulse reaction as a warning sign of a life-threatening crisis and the lasting remedying of the crisis.
- Procedures that influence and measure increases and decreases in arterial and venous O_2 blood levels.
- The necessary physical exercise to attain a training effect (which is less than you might expect).
- Increases in brain circulation during physical strain.

- Rate of blood flow in the circulation of the organs.
- Various examples in changes of O_2 uptake. Heart minute volume and blood flow of the organs decisive for O_2 transport.
- Relation of ATP concentrations in rat brains as a function of the oxygen partial pressure of the inspired air.

von Ardenne graphed much of his research. Other co-factors that influence lung volume include: airways hyper-responsiveness, atopy, childhood respiratory infections, air pollution, posture, subluxation of the spine, exercise, deep and superficial fascia, nutrition, occupational hazards, abuse and trauma, attitude, and age, height, weight and sex.

MORE BREATHING CO-FACTORS

In a recent **Health Sciences Institute** newsletter, major medical journals confirmed that simple breathing techniques could reduce blood pressure, treat asthma and eliminate pain.

Breathe away disease without drugs, surgery or even supplements! Squash heart disease and hypertension...
Strike out irritable bowel and ulcers... Eliminate arthritis, gout and back pain...Beat insomnia and stressed out nerves... Ease menstrual and menopausal suffering...Clobber asthma and bronchitis...

Suddenly, strangely, all manner of "incurable" ailments are literally vanishing into thin air...!

Imagine your blood pressure plummeting in minutes...
Simply breathing away the pain when your arthritis flares up...
Instantly calming colitis, even if you've been suffering all your life...
Feeling hot flashes fade away, without the need for HRT.

- ✘ Do you experience shallow, labored breathing; shortness of breath; a high chest; stuck, erratic, or reverse breathing?
- ✘ Are you unable to catch your breath?
- ✘ Do you have blue-tinted lips or fingernails; trouble sleeping;
- ✘ Do you have more than 4-5 resting breaths per minute with

3-6 second pauses; heart beat irregularities; poor posture, mild to severe depression; tightness across your chest; excessive stress; asthma or COPD symptoms; constant fatigue; chronic pain; chest pains; anger; anxiety; hyperventilation?
✘ Do you often catch yourself not breathing?
✘ Do you think you can't sing or want to sing better?

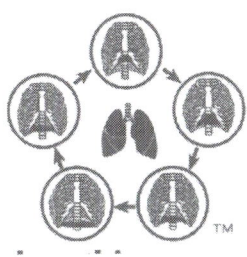

For more breathing-relevant studies in a free newsletter or take our FREE breathing self-tests and see how you compare to others, go to:
http://www.breathing.com/tests.htm

Breathing properly will oxygenate the body but it also may well balance the nervous system. In other words, given even pristine circumstances on ALL levels of nutrition, environment, toxicity, exterior stresses and all other factors influencing the human condition, the nervous system will never be or stay balanced without balanced breathing.

Traditional respiratory models often over-use drugs and surgery. Breathing mechanics and respiration are compromised long before they are detected by conventional diagnosis. Asthma, bronchitis, laryngitis, emphysema, COPD, Spasmodic Dysphonia, stuttering, panic disorders and heart conditions all have HUGE breathing components, do not develop overnight and often take decades to develop enough to become "symptoms". By that time the patient has lost over 50% of their breathing function!

People with poor oxygen levels, lessened brain function, compromised cellular strength, hampered detoxification and overworked nervous systems develop sickness or "symptoms" more often and stay sick longer.

Go to the Free Breathing Tests at http://www.breathing.com/tests.htm for an in depth assessment of your breathing

Identifying Causes of Unbalanced Dysfunctional Breathing (UDB) Gives You A Starting Point for Rebuilding Your Health!

"Breathing is the FIRST place not the LAST place one should investigate when any disordered energy presents itself."
— Sheldon Saul Hendler, MD Ph.D. *The Oxygen Breakthrough*

DIAPHRAGM DEVELOPMENT – Your primary muscle organ for breathing.

From an enlightened medical doctor..."Mr. A had an injury to his diaphragm -- inability to function properly --adversely affecting his breathing. There is no established medical treatment for this condition and patient has been encouraged to seek any and all alternative treatment modalities." Partly good advice but yikes on the many sources of mediocre to bad information sources that are out in the world these days. We begin with the 176Video/ DVD and diaphragm strengthener. Everything else centers around this extremely powerful 1-2 combination.

Your diaphragm is a prime mediator of all the biological and emotional rhythms of your body. Including the autonomic nervous system including brain functions of circadian and ultradian rhythms. The rhythmic movement of your diaphragm is changing constantly. It is shaped like a half dome arching into the cavity of your chest. As you inhale it contracts down pressing on your organs and hopefully with a proper deep breath, opens up your chest. Air comes in as you breathe in and goes out as you exhale. During the exhale your diaphragm relaxes and rises like the handle on a bicycle pump being withdrawn up so it's ready to draw air into your lungs.

Your diaphragm shrinks and weakens as you age. Your "bicycle pump" (diaphragm) gets smaller and can't draw as much air as it did when you were in your 20's and 30's.. As it ages, your diaphragm loses some or most of its nervous-system-balancing-ability. This means you can and should learn how much of so-called diaphragmatic breathing really ISN'T full breathing at all!

Poor breathing is a cause and contributor to most disease and nervous system dysfunction. Make absolutely sure you develop your breathing by using our exercises shown on the #176 Video/DVD and the Optimal Diaphragm Strengthener: http://www.breathing.com/video-ds.htm and sometimes the Blue Velcro Strap: http://www.breathing.com/bvs.htm

CHAPTER 1
Mechanical Breathing Function

Breathing mechanics and respiration will oxygenate the body but they may also balance or unbalance the nervous system. In other words, given pristine circumstances on ALL levels of nutrition, environment, toxicity, exterior stresses and all other factors influencing the human condition, the nervous system will never be or stay balanced without the ease, depth and balance of one's breathing.

Traditional respiratory models often over-use drugs and surgery. Breathing mechanics and respiration are compromised long before they are detected by conventional diagnosis. Asthma, Bronchitis, laryngitis, Emphysema, COPD, Spasmodic dysphonia, stuttering, panic disorders and heart conditions which all have HUGE breathing components do not develop overnight and often take decades to present. By that time the patient has lost over 50% of their breathing function.

People who have poor oxygen levels, lessened brain function, compromised cellular strength, hampered detoxification and overworked nervous systems get sick more often and stay sick longer.

Unbalanced or undetected Dysfunctional Breathing (UDB) is both a cause and contributor to most disease.

Breathing mechanics and respiration will oxygenate the body but they may also balance or unbalance the nervous system. In other words, given pristine circumstances on ALL levels of nutrition, environment, toxicity, exterior stresses and all other factors influencing the human condition, the nervous system will never be or stay balanced without the ease, depth and balance of one's breathing.

Traditional respiratory models often over-use drugs and surgery. **Breathing mechanics and respiration are compromised long before they are detected by conventional diagnosis.** Asthma, bronchitis, laryngitis, Emphysema, COPD, Spasmodic dysphonia, stuttering, panic disorders and heart conditions all have HUGE breathing components and do not develop overnight. They often take <u>decades</u> to present. **By that time the patient has often lost over 50% of their breathing function!**

People with poor oxygen levels, lessened brain function, compromised cellular strength, hampered detoxification and overworked nervous systems get sick more often and stay sick longer.

Assessing for UDB is fairly simple. Go to <u>http://www.breathing.com/tests.htm</u> and take our FREE Breathing Tests. There are over 100 test factors presented that allude to the following page of UDB cofactors. Take the free breathing tests to see how much your breathing might be impacting or impacted by the following UDB list.

Unbalanced Dysfunctional Breathing - UDB

UDB causes or increases shortness of breath, hyperventilation, anxiety, panic attacks, seizures, asthma, COPD, nervous system dysfunction, etc. Bad breathing can: *make you anxious *make you sick/sicker *make you think you're crazy *destroy your energy *make/keep you fat *steal your personal power *hinder your voice and *shorten your life. Your breathing may be "authentic" but still severely unbalanced. **Make copies of this page so you can record your progress for 3-6 months.** Or download our PDF file to keep on file. http://www.breathing.com/articles/udb.htm Check (✔) the numbers (issues) you're experiencing now. **At subsequent evaluations, report good progress or where you feel you need to improve or change what you're doing.** Close your eyes, go within and inhale and exhale deeply (twice), as you would normally breathe. Open your eyes and reflect on whether you (now or often) experience any of these issues. More than two circles means you are experiencing UDB.

Breath is life! *Improve your breathing NOW !!*

1. Addicted
2. Air hunger
3. Allergies
4. Altitude makes breathing harder
5. Anxiety –chronic
   5b. Anger –chronic
   5c Fear - chronic
6. Apathy
7. Apnea
8. Attention problems
9. Back pain–low or mid back
10. Bluish cast to lips, nail beds
11. Bowel or rectum disorder
12. Blood sugar swings (wide)
13. Look in a mirror and breathe as deeply as you can. Do your neck muscles bulge out? Your shoulders or collarbones rise?
14. Breathing feels like a series of events, instead of one smooth internally coordinated continuous flow
15. Breathing feels stuck
16. Breath heaving
17. Breathing labored/restricted
18. Breathing is shallow
19. Breathlessness
20. Can't catch breath or deep breathing curtailed
21. Can't feel breath in nostrils
22. Can't meditate
23. Can't relax
24. Can't sleep on back
25. Can't walk and easily talk at the same time
26. Chest is large and stiff
27. Chest pain
28. Chest sunken
29. Chest tightness after surgery
30. Chest wall defects (faults)
31. Chest wall tenderness
32. Chronic cough
33. Chronic pain
34. Cold hands or sweaty palm
35. Cold temp bothers breathing
36. Confrontations make your voice pitch go up
37. Confused or sense of losing normal contact with surroundings
38. Constant fatigue
39. Constipation
40. Cramps in abdomen or below sternum, or side stitches
41. Depression
42. Digestion poor

42b. Ulcer
43. Diaphragm excursion poor
44. Diaphragmatic impairment
45. Dizzy when excited-anxious
46. Do you often PRESS your tongue to the roof of your mouth?
47. Dry mouth
48. Fanny sticks out in rear
49. Fall asleep watching TV or at theater when you would rather watch program?
50. Feel a hitch, bump or lump right below your breastbone when you try to take a deep breath
51. Feelings of suffocation
52. Finish other's sentences for them
53. Furrows brow often
54. Gasping
55. Get tired from reading out loud?
56. Get drowsy from driving a vehicle
57. Grind teeth at night
58. Dynamic hyperinflation
59. Headaches
60. Heart condition or attack(s)
61. Heavy breathing
62. High blood pressure
63. History of or present lung disease
64. History of abuse or trauma
65. Hold breath a lot
66. Hormonal fluctuations
67. Hot flashes
68. Hyperventilation, over-breathing
69. Hypocapnea (exhale too little carbon dioxide)
70. Hypoglycemia
71. Irregular heartbeats
72. Irregularly formed rib cage (can you see it in mirror?)
73. Jaw tension
74. Jet lag or severe jet lag
75. Longevity wanted
76. Lump in throat
77. Migraines
78. Mouth breather
79. Nightmares
80. Nodules
81. Obese
82. Often catch yourself not breathing?
83. Often shift weight from side to side while standing
84. Panic attacks
85. People have difficulty hearing you and are not partly deaf
86. Phobic
87. Poor boundaries
88. Poor sleep
89. Posture poor
90. Pregnant
91. Public speaking
92. Pulsing or stabbing feeling in and around ribs
93. Reduced pain tolerance
94. Reflux
95. Repetitive strain injury
96. Ribs flair outward at bottom during inhale
97. Sallow complexion
98. Scoliosis or abnormal curvature of the spine
99. Seizures
100. Self esteem poor
101. Shortness of breath
102. Shortened stride
103. Shoulders rounded forward
104. Sigh or yawn often
105. Singing poorly
106. Snore
107. Soreness or pain in throat with "prolonged" vocal use
108. Sore deep pain feels like a band across your chest
109. Speech problems
110. Sports/exercise induced asthma
111. Stiff neck
112. Stressed out
113. Stomach tense while unaware or unable to relax it.
114. Stroke
115. Sunken chest
116. Sustaining low tones difficult
117. Swallowing difficulty
118. Swim - can't at all, as well or as easily as you used to
119. Talking on the phone makes you short of breath
120. Tension around the eyes
121. Tense overall feeling (hypertension)
122. Thoughts run amuck
123. Tightness around mouth
124. Thoracic insufficiency syndrome

125. Tightness, soreness or pressure in the chest or below breast bone
126. Type "A" personality
127. Upper note singin problems
128. Upset stomach or irritable bowel syndrome
129. Vision blurred or eyesight better in AM than beforebed?
130. Voice or speech problem
131. Voice feels weak
132. Nervous quiver in voice
133. Wake from sleep suddenly not breathing = Apnea
134. Washboard abs
135. Wake up tired a lot
136. Wheezing

My breathing is mainly ____
(SH)=Shallow; (L)=Labored;
(F)=Fast; (SL)=Slow
(D)=Deep, (B)=Belly
(HC)=High Chest
(CO)=Cough; (HB)=Hold breath;
(E)=Erratic

UDB© or Unbalanced Dysfunctional Breathing© was first clarified by Michael G. White, Optimal Breathing® Coach. It's wise to eliminate UDB as it can severely hinder oxygenation and nervous system function. More about this at http://www.breathing.com/articles/udb.htm and http://www.breathing.com/articles/carbon-dioxide.htm

Optimal Breathing® Toll Free 866 My Inhale
866.694.6425
© 2004 Michael Grant White

CHAPTER 2
Posture & Ergonomics

FIRST COMES THE DIAPHRAGM.
Redevelopment of the diaphragm is the primary goal of **Optimal Breathing**®. The lungs are quite important but secondary in terms of development. As the diaphragm shrinks it will rise less and less up into the chest and allow the lungs to build up "debris" in the form of bacteria and toxins.

Compare the function of the diaphragm to a bicycle pump. If you pull the pump handle out just a little you get very little air into the tire when you push the plunger in or down. As the pump handle rises so does the diaphragm rise and similarly the more air it can pull into the lungs. Due to poor usage, the diaphragm can shrink and weaken. A larger higher rise /excursion is better than being only stronger because if the diaphragm rise is larger it will also be stronger, but if it is stronger it may not be larger. Breathing VOLUME is the key to optimal oxygenation and longevity.

Think of the diaphragm as a face-down half-dome-shaped bowl (like a fresh halved plum) resting downward on the flattened surface. Imagine its sides weakening and shriveling up all around like a prune. This means that the diaphragm is affected on ALL sides of it. Poor posture such as slouching or tilting sideways can cause it to be unable to rise or expand outwardly. This restriction of full rise and fall (excursion) can weaken any part of its bowl shaped surface. Since it's a muscle, the diaphragm most often stays weakened unless something is done about it. The ancient saying "if you don't use it you lose it " is very appropriate here!

When the diaphragm shrinks it often shrinks irregularly. This happens with almost every lung issue. I had a video fluoroscopes of MY diaphragm. It was fascinating. The MD radiologist was kind enough to let me x-ray my diaphragm but did not have a protocol for this, which suggests to me a lack of clinical research into diaphragm function and development.

Try this. Sit down and bend over and try to breathe in. Notice how it is harder to breathe. This is an extreme example of how our muscles and tendons get over restricted and cause a reduction of depth and ease of breathing.

SIT UP STRAIGHT?

People are often asked to sit up straight. This rarely has permanent effect because by the time someone needs to be reminded to do so, their body has adapted to being more comfortable in the slouching position. When they attempt to sit up "straight" they actually tighten the already over-shortened frontal muscles and tendons, and this causes restrictions in the ease of breathing volume. Tightening these muscles even more to make oneself more erect causes tightness in the entire upper body and reduces the ease of deep breathing. We intuitively do not like this and soon adjust back to where it was easier to breathe.

That's why most people who are advised to sit up straight, remain erect for only a few minutes before reverting to their former slouch where breathing was easier. Their breathing is still held back from being fully deep, easy and balanced. For them it's easier and what they've become accustomed to. Often what we perceive as satisfactory is a lack of adequate understanding. Extreme examples of this are called delusions.

Sitting for long periods of time are good opportunities to cause shortened frontal muscles. Lots of computer time, desk jockeying or vehicle driving help (see video 176 and 191 manual for specific ways to modify or purchase office, airplane, home and car seating) create the posture that makes for semi-permanent shallow breathing. Many easy chairs and airplane seats invite suppressed breathing.

To repeat, you cannot HOLD yourself upright to achieve optimal breathing. By the time you might benefit from that, the muscles in the front of your body have become over-shortened from slouching and over-lengthened in the back. Making the body more erect actually shortens those already too short muscles in the front. This causes a lessening of ease in breathing volume, and reduces the ease of deeper breathing; we intuitively do not like that. That is why most people remain erect only for a few minutes before reverting to their usual slouch.

Bodywork such a Rolfing or myofacial massage can help but it is the moment-to-moment feedback of internal sensing, feeling and movement of the optimal breathing that is most beneficial.

SUBTLE SIGNALS
Poor posture causes or is a result of tensions in various parts of the body. If your knees or pelvis are locked up they block off energy flowing up and down your body, including your spine. This reduces the depth of your easy breathing. Try standing perfectly balanced in both legs for 5 natural effortless breaths. Adjust your weight placing more weight on one leg (wait 5 breaths), then both legs (wait 5 breaths) then the other leg (wait for 5 breaths) and experience the breathing going less deep and easy as you transfer your weight into one leg or the other. Even this seemingly insignificant "posture" restricts your ease and depth of breathing and eventually your energy.

ATTITUDE
What ever your posture at any given moment in time, it's influencing your breathing and attitude. It's often easy to spot someone with a distorted or negative attitude by their slumped shoulders, bent over, weak-kneed and hang-dog posture.

Posture often shapes and forms attitude. Attitude can help create good or bad posture.

BENT OVER POSTURE
Poor posture restricts the rise and fall of the breathing diaphragm. We also know from chiropractors that an overly bent or unbalanced spine restricts vital life force. Nerve force energy restrictions in the spine mean less life force into all the major organs fed by the spinal nerves, including your heart, lungs and brain. So now we have lessened nerve force in addition to reduced ease and depth of natural oxygenation and *nervous system* un-*balance* stemming from restricted or unbalanced breathing.

Have you ever noticed that people who sit up straight seem to be more alert? They ARE!

ROUNDED SHOULDERS

Rounded shoulders restrict the expansion of the rib cage, diaphragm rise and lung volume. Forcing the shoulders back and the body to remain erect improves the situation somewhat but again, also tightens up those same problem rib, torso and neck muscles and restricts the deepest, easiest breathing. Great techniques and exercises to offset rounded shoulders are in the 176 video/DVD.

Observe these pictures for extreme examples of negative posturing and tensions.

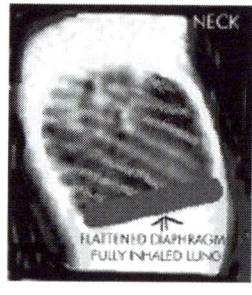

#1. Fully Inhaled Lung

#1 full inhale (left). The chest is flat or slightly rounded outwardly. Notice there is usually more lung tissue in the back of the torso than in the front. But due to poor posture it's less easily accessed.

Note the exhaled, inward curve of the chest in **#2 full exhale** (right) with the lungs 7-C above greatly emptied. When we exhale, the lungs and chest naturally collapse and less air is inside us. The lungs have no muscle and are almost passive, so when we breathe in again the ribs must allow for expansion of the lungs to the fullest. This allows the diaphragm to draw in the deepest, fullest breath. But the diaphragm must be of sufficient size (not strength) to draw in the maximum air.

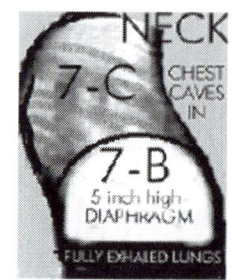

#2. Fully Exhaled Lung

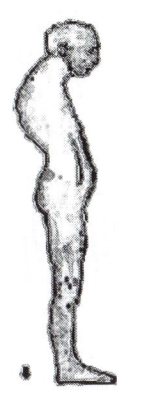

#3 Slouching

In **#3 Slouching** (left) the upper chest posture has collapsed, creating more of the shape of the completely expired lung in **#1**. Lungs with little or no air left. Only this person hasn't exhaled. They are trying to breathe but have difficulty doing so. Variations of this are experienced as Unbalanced deep Breathing - UDB.

LOOKING DOWNWARD TOO OFTEN

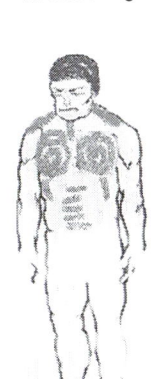

When you look downward you only see what's on the ground — more importantly, your body adapts to being bent over. This also limits natural vision (eye exercising) which should have a wide variety of depth and color. When you limit what you see, you limit your moment-to-moment experience. Looking downward may be helpful for "deep thought" but it produces a negative outcome on your posture and attitude.

#4 (left) shows an overly muscled upper body that cannot easily expand. Stomach, chest and shoulder muscles are like the body of a man needing to carry or pull heavy loads and slouch slightly all the while. When the muscles set in cement he never gets to set the load down. His ribcage ALWAYS stays stiff and inflexible. A heart attack, lung disease or malady caused from shortness of oxygen is waiting to happen.

In her book *"Posture, Getting it Straight"* Janice Novak states that good posture can add up to ten years to your life. I suggest it's many more YEARS than that. The QUALITY of your breathing determines your longevity!

In my *Secrets of Optimal Natural Breathing* manual you will see more examples of diaphragm development and posture relationships and how they compromise the ability to fully breathe; plus simple ways to ensure you develop your posture to help develop and maintain your Optimal Breathing.

AWARENESS

One needs to rapidly open up the breathing to make it larger and in balance and with that you become more apt to notice changes from moment to moment. If you go too slowly or too quickly you miss many opportunities for progress.

REMEMBER

You can't HOLD yourself upright to achieve optimal breathing because the muscles in the front of your body have become over-shortened front to back, side to side and in rotation from slouching. These muscles have also been over-lengthened in the back from the same slouching. Slouching also develops weakened abdominal or over-tight back muscles. You need to develop internal coordination and posture, from the inside out. The easiest and most effective and lasting way to develop coordination is to develop É moment to moment............ your breathing.

Nada Chair

WHEEL CHAIRS

cause most people to slouch and round their shoulders, causing shallow, unbalanced breathing. Develop your breathing as well as look into getting a Nada Chair (http://www.breathing.com/nada.htm). Excellent posture is indispensable to proper breathing. For the diaphragm to rise its highest the chest must be open with the ribs raised out of the way and the body erect or prone, never bent at any angle front side or back. That means that every thing we sit or recline in must support the way we breathe.

All **Optimal Breathing**® is diaphragmatic +lower rib breathing. Some people with COPD do breathe diaphragmatically, just not very much. They utilize practically NO lower rib breathing. Most people who develop COPD tend to breathe with the upper ribs and hardly any diaphragm. We need BOTH.

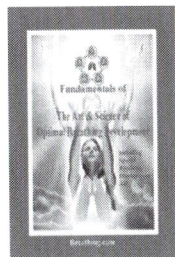

While using the exercises demonstrated on our **#176 DVD** and the Diaphragm Strengthener (http://www.breathing.com/video-ds.htm), you can address these problems by making the breathing larger and smoother and easier. When breathing is proper, you will be quick to notice the difference when you do things that make breathing volume smaller, restricting your breathing, making it harder to breathe fully and deeply. Poor posture is the major cause.

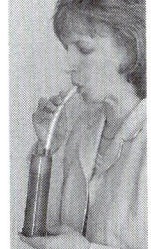

CHAPTER 3.
MOVEMENT AND LUNG FUNCTION

Movement is an indispensable catalyst to digestion, elimination, circulation and respiration!

MOST PEOPLE DO N'T MOVE ENOUGH!
The lungs require expansion and contraction to stay clean and functional. The rib cage must open and close with each deep breath. Regardless of diet, excessive shallow or distorted breathing will invite a host of bacteria and environmental debris. The diaphragm also needs to be large and strong, but will not be large if the rib cage does not expand. A small and strong diaphragm is not nearly as oxygen-producing as a LARGE and strong diaphragm.

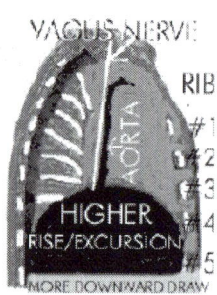 To strengthen the diaphragm is very important, but not as important as size and excursion (rise... see graphic on left). The larger the rise the stronger the diaphragm becomes. 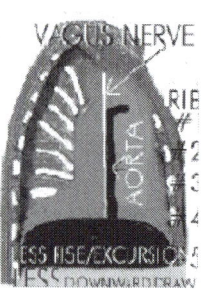 **Rise = movement. Just like an elevator.** The diaphragm interconnects your abdomen, lungs and spine. **Because of these relationships diaphragm movement is profoundly influenced by posture.**

Posture is critical, however, as soon as someone with poor posture sits up straight the muscles in the front of the body that are too short and cause the slouching get tighter and shorter and that suppresses deeper, easier breathing. People intuitively do not care for that feeling and soon go back to slouching, because in that body position it was a little easier to for them to breathe. Most do not have a clue about that aspect of their breathing and suffer because of their lack of awareness. Video flourescopy can show you exactly how high the diaphragm is rising. The number count in the Free Breathing tests is our non-scientific way to simultaneously gauge diaphragm rise and exhale efficiency.

Tai chi, gentle Yoga, dance (I love to Tango) movement therapy, low impact aerobics, T5T, Butoh and anything that gently gets you off your butt can do wonders for circulation and mobility. We have created several programs in the Secrets of Optimal Breathing® Manual that gets you moving and breathing. If you already do something you like, then stick with it and vary how you're moving, making sure you also develop good breathing fundamentals.

Some people find it difficult to get up and move. This may well be a breathing issue. They do not have the juice to get the juice is the way I often put it. If you have worked with our **#176 DVD/ video "Fundamentals" program** (right) and still are not wanting to get-up-and-go, then you better look into the other factors discussed in this book. Also consider oxygen generators and Far Infrared saunas purchased at a deep discount at our programs page (http://www.breathing.com/sauna.htm) and come to our Optimal Breathing School (http://www.breathing.com/school/main.htm)

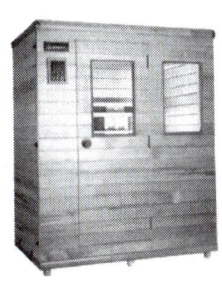
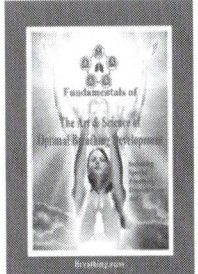

Many people have lost their kinesthetic /proprioceptiveness (physical sensing and feeling) — what their breathing feels like.

They do not move enough. Mobile trainees need be reminded daily what is needed to "feel" the way they're breathing. Bedridden people must be visited daily and trained by professionals or loved ones until it's clear they won't digress — even then they must be reminded daily to move and breathe right at the same time.

Volunteers can be trained to help with daily reminders for proper breathing maintenance. Extremely difficult cases may take six months or more, but I believe most people can be walking and smiling again in due time and without drugs or surgery. For patients with lung disease, a recumbent stationary bike or mobile tricycle can help. Their head and neck must be supported and the chest "opened" so the breather doesn't activate "accessory" (constricting) breathing muscles in the neck and torso and close off some of the "easier" inhaled air supply.

I also recommend swimming with a mask, fins and snorkel in warm water (85 - 95 degrees) in a *face down position*. The mask, fins and snorkel will allow the person to relax and breathe in slight "extension" or backward bending enough to open the chest for easier breathing. The breaststroke or backstroke is best because these strokes open the chest.

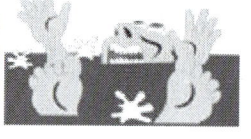

Combining an oxygen generator with some sort of treadmill or stationary bicycle can help a great deal. Mistakes I have observed in many pulmonary rehab units are being addressed at our Optimal Breathing School (http://www.breathing.com/school/main.htm).

ORGANS, NERVOUS SYSTEM AND DIAPHRAGM FUNCTION

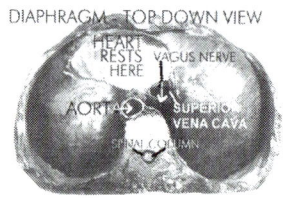

The heart rests on top of the diaphragm. The liver, gall bladder spleen, stomach and kidneys lie below it. These organs are massaged significantly - to the degree that the diaphragm moves fully up and down. Your diaphragm is attached to your spine and rib cage and moves (or not) with the movements of those vetebra and ribs. As the ribs and spine move they transfer muscle tightening and releasing that influences the volume, rise and descent of the diaphragm.

DANCING AND BREATHING

I'm probably going to get some static from this — but it has been my observation, as well as colleague Joni Wilson (http://www.joniwilsonvoice.com), that dancers are often very poor breathers. Most dancing requires quick or extreme movements and breathing suffers. Many of the muscles that need to let go during breathing must contract during dancing. Most yoga is definitely not the answer either as too many yoga teachers have a strange way of using the breathing stemming from the "complete breath", where the belly goes in on the exhale.

Stretching can be very helpful. To be clearer about this, you will never see a major opera singer who is also a major dancer. Fred Astaire was a great dancer, but only a mediocre singerÉ Gene Kelly and Donald O'Conner as well. One dance that seems to be more breathing-friendly is the Argentine TangoÉ but that greatly depends on the way the teacher addresses breathing. I've seen a few tango teachers who obviously have no idea what **Optimal Breathing**® looks, FEELS or acts like.

Tango and Tai Chi seem to have much in common — when taught from a better respect and care for the breathing process. One thing dancers must avoid is the tendency to allow their neck muscles to bulge out during dancing or movement. Practice nose breathe as well. It's most always best. There must be many other dances or movement expression styles that favor breathing such as Butoh (to me it is about freedom) or even contra dancing. Mind the neck muscles, since they are indicators of activation of accessory breathing muscles and possible future breathing and voice issues.

Energy increases exponentially as you utilize the exercises on our **#176Video/ DVD** and the **Diaphragm Strengthener** (http://www.breathing.com/video-ds.htm). Movement produces increased flow and energy!

CHAPTER 4.
BREATHING EXERCISES

It is rather unusual to many of us in the western world to consider the importance of breathing techniques or breathing development After all, we are always breathing, aren't we? It seems a little silly to put extra attention to something we do naturally. Notice your own breathing. Isn't each breath actually very shallow?

The magnitude of the crisis in modern medicine demands immediate and broadly pervasive consumer action to enhance health and curb medical spending. Simply put — appropriate breathing development, practiced vigilantly and on a daily basis, can precipitate an absolutely remarkable revolution in our personal lives as well as influence the history of human health care and medical evolution.

The presence of special breathing practices in the ancient cultures has always been a mystery to people in the Western world. There are numerous beneficial physiological mechanisms that are triggered when we turn our attention to the breath and then increase it's ease, depth, volume and balance.
When breathing volume, rate, balance and awareness are all optimized, dramatic physiological, and even emotional, changes can occur. As it turns out, unknown to science until very recently, the action of the lungs, diaphragm and thorax are a primary pump for the lymph fluid and heart as well as a huge influence in keeping the Autonomic Nervous System in balance. In addition, the breath is the primary source for oxygen, which is the key element in the body's ability to produce energy.

However, *"To actually transform our breathing and bring about a lasting change, the reeducation exercises we do must be based on the laws and principles of natural breathing, and must be done in such a way that the body/mind can either "re-member" these laws or learn them anew,"* says Dennis Lewis, author of **The Tao of Natural Breathing**.

Just because one particular breathing exercise or breathing technique feels good doesn't mean it's healthy or will resolve a breathing development goal, or result in a long-term aid in a wellness or performance program. Just because one particular breathing exercise or breathing technique feels good does not mean it is healthy or will resolve a breathing development goal or result in a long-term aid in a wellness or performance program.

Our **Optimal Breathing® Development System** is not so much about breathing exercises. We employ a few exercises, but we've learned that "breathing exercises" mean many things to many people and as a grouping is a potpourri of good, mediocre, bad, confusing and outright dangerously unhealthy ways for using the breath and breathing.

We carefully choose what breathing exercises we DO employ, based upon physical function, form and the health, peak performance, self-expression, emotional balance and life extension goals of our students. Patients and people with performance or personal development goals who have learned and used a proper breathing development practice as a part of their daily personal system progress quicker, no matter what their health or performance goals. Individuals who are well are able to remain healthier, adapt to greater stress and have greater endurance when they keep a breathing development practice in their daily self-care ritual.

Altered states of consciousness are huge aspect of many breathing exercises. I have seen many of those altered states turn into erratic or weird behavior including what was classified as psychosis.

We have created several popular training program sets. (http://www.breathing.com/programs.htm) These programs are comprehensive, easy to learn, easy to apply, require no special knowledge or training and many can be practiced in varying degrees by all people (sick or well) daily with very little impact on time or energy. Many of the self-help versions can be successfully learned without a teacher present. In fact, they actually give the individual, both time and energy, because there is less cost, fatigue, and forgetfulness, because the function of the organs and glands is enhanced and regenerated. They are a great way to recharge your cellular batteries.

Every minute spent applying the techniques in our **Optimal Breathing® System** is returned (to the practitioner) as a need for less sleep.

Every unit of energy spent brings forth an internal ability to generate an even greater amount of energy!

With the recent "new age" popularity of daily conscious breathing exercises, many people are being trained to either breathe into the belly, consistently watch their breath, create postures that are supposed to expand the breathing (many do, some don't), or forcefully inhale or exhale in an attempt to increase breathing rate or volume.

The belly breath can stabilize the nervous systems and emotions and is generally a good place to begin breathing development. However, I've seen many exceptions to this because an improperly trained belly breath can also become an habitual distraction and breathing restriction. It is also just a beginning.

Watching the breath is helpful for many people to focus and get calm, however, it can also develop into an on-going distraction. Postures can expand or distribute the breath, as well as cause the breathing restriction they hope to eliminate. The forcefulness/ effort can be valuable, but is, in many ways, unnecessary and can cause sympathetic arousal and restriction of full breathing volume, i.e. "breathing blocks". These blocks are tensions and postures in the body that restrict the natural flow of the breathing energy called life-force, chi, ki, qi, ha, prana, pneuma, elan vital, etc.

Breathing awareness, physical assessments and sound production quality and quantity are the primary markers for positive change of the breath.

EASIER, FULLER, LONG TERM BREATHING IMPROVEMENT?

Many techniques exist to modify, direct or observe the activity of breathing. Each has its purpose and limitation. Any one exercise you do with the breath will, after enough repetitions, restrict the diaphragm and rib cage's freedom and fullness. When you forcibly take deeper belly breaths you also partially stimulate the sympathetic nervous system because you are "efforting the activity."

When practicing breath awareness, your observation of the breath may cause it to speed up, slow down or become shallow. Several clients told me that trying to follow their breath made them extremely anxious, and others just couldn't do it due to stress and internal distractions. This is, to me, an indicator of UDB.

Optimal breath awareness develops more from skill levels such as coordinated singing, speaking, walking and movement oriented activities. When you utilize the exercises on our **#176Video/ DVD** and **Diaphragm Strengthener** everything else works better (http://www.breathing.com/video-ds.htm) breathing exercises, nutrition, cleansing, detoxification — everything!

CHAPTER 5.
The Squeeze and Breathe Technique

MIKE'S FAVORITE: The Squeeze and Breathe Technique

© 2004 All rights reserved. http://www.breathing.com/squeezeandbreathe.htm

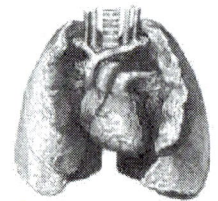

There are many breathing exercises. For most people, there may be only *one* really good exercise that works *well* as a starting point to guide someone with poor to very poor breathing. The best exercise(es) either energize or slow down/calm the breathing, or both. What's *optimal* also increases breathing volume and therefore one's longevity.

The following breathing exercise will help do ALL three: slowing, energizing and expanding. Good endorphin production seems to stem from a strong parasympathetic/relaxing breathing pattern. When done properly, this exercise increases significant energy, as well as relaxation.

Anxiety can be caused (or stress increased) by poor breathing speed and erratic/unbalanced sequencing. This exercise is very good for reducing anxiety and/or depression. Extreme forms of emotion are often immobilizing, limiting and dangerous to one's health and well-being. Emotions can be deadly. Anxiety can harm and even kill. The way you breathe can reduce or increase your emotional/fear response.

Look at the lungs above (cut back to show how the heart fits into that space). Notice how the lungs are smaller at the top. This means it's pointless to breathe into the high chest because there's very little lung volume there.

The mid chest and lower rear lung lobes are where the major breathing volume is obtained (the back of the trunk from mid back to waist). This area allows the most expansion. Tension in the low back tends to restrict expansion, so we must both access and challenge that area in the following way.

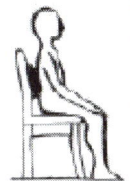

For breathing that is quieting, calming, centering and energizing all at once: Stand with knees slightly bent is preferable with tail bone tilted gently forward. Or Supported by a small round pillow (at left) or use a NADA Chair (on right), http://www.breathing.com/nada.htm sit near the front edge of a fairly hard surfaced chair, stool or arm of a couch, with your feet flat on the floor. Both of these positions need an erect but not stiff posture. Stand or sit "tallest" with your chin even with (or above) the horizon and gently tucked in.

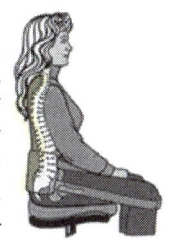

NADA Chair

If you stand, bend your knees slightly to unlock them.
Lightly touch your tongue to the roof of your mouth and let your jaw relax. Relax your belly. Let it hang down. Let go of any thought of having a "pot belly" or not having "wash- board abs".

Place your thumbs over your kidneys (below your back ribs and above your pelvis - (photo #1 at left). Wrap your fingers around your sides towards your belly button (as if you are getting a front-to-back firm grip on "love handles" - or that general area). Get a good grip by squeezing your fingers and thumbs together firmly, then breathe through your nose (a long, slow, deep 3-count in-breath). Force your squeezed fingers (Photo #2) apart with your in-breath, against the tension in your squeezed fingers. (Use the force of breathing-in to make your fingers and thumbs expand.)

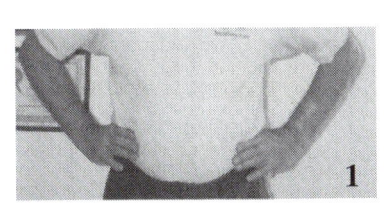

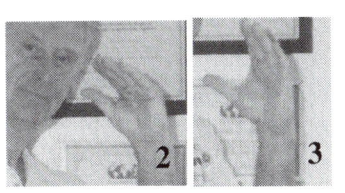

Then relax your grip (Photo #3) and slow down the exhale so it lasts for a count of seven (7). Never tighten the belly to extend the exhale. Simply slow the speed of the out-breath. Always keep the belly relaxed.

Do this exercise again, use a 3-count inhale and 7-count exhale. If you did not feel better from this exercise, we encourage you to take our Free Breathing Tests and see why and how to develop your breathing: http://www.breathing.com/tests.htm

HOW DID IT FEEL?

Dizziness, spacey ness, or confusion or anxiety means you:
A. Probably did not squeeze in the right place – like on the bone of the pelvis or ribs   or squeeze or did not squeeze hard enough.
B. Or you breathed too fast. SLOW down the exhale by adding 3-7 counts to the exhale and try it again in one minute.
C. Wait a minute or two, after the energy has subsided or integrated within you and do   it again.
D. Still anxious or dizzy or both? - You may have severe UDB - in which case you should stop and call us for a recommendation.
E. You REALLY need to learn this!

Did it FEEL relaxing, energizing? Are you calmer? Energized?

Calm and energized at the same time? Anxious? If anxious, try to lengthen the exhale count, while keeping the inhale count the same or smaller. Example: a 3 count inhale and 10 count exhale or 3 count inhale and 12 count exhale.

A 20 count exhale should eventually be attainable, but for some people it might take weeks or months to develop. (Remember: NEVER tighten your belly to make the exhale last longer.) Just let the air out slower. You should eventually feel a calming and energizing effect throughout your entire body.

If that is not the right feel or timing, then experiment with the same inhales, but longer or shorter exhales, until you discover a comfortable pattern that you can repeat.

The Squeeze & Breathe Technique[a] is very effective but still temporary approach to breathing development. It is the prelude to using the 176Video/DVD and Diaphragm Strengthener and sometimes the Blue Velcro Strap. http://www.breathing.com/video-ds.htm   http://www.breathing.com/video-bvs-ds.htm

Chapter 6.
Diet and Nutrition

START EATING MORE ORGANIC RAW LIVING FOODS
"Our local news station this week ran a story that showed that certain areas of the brain are stimulated when one peels an apple. The area of the brain that lit up on the scan was an area most often devoted to higher-level thinking/problem-solving. It got me thinking. Just imagine... if cutting and peeling an apple does this much good for our brain, IMAGINE how much positive juice is flowing to our brains on a raw food diet (cutting and preparing all kinds of good fruits and veggies, etc...)!!!"
Deborah (raw egroup)
Right on Deborah!

GENETICALLY MODIFIED FOODS
GM crops are becoming more and more prevalent, and the spread of GM seeds and pollen is a major concern. Even organic products may be contaminated with traces of GM elements that have been spread by wind or insects such as bees. Eating organic is currently the best way to ensure that your food has not been genetically modified. By definition, food that is certified organic must be: free from all GM organisms; produced without artificial pesticides and fertilizers; from an animal reared without the routine use of antibiotics, growth promoters or other drugs.

FEEDING YOUR LUNGS
"No other animals on the planet find it hard to eat raw foods – just brainwashed humansÉ!"
— **Jan Jenson**, The WELL-th Coach!

Start following the lives of people like David Wolf, Victoras Kulvinskas, Doug Graham, Paul Bragg, Norman Walker, David Klein, and Jan Jenson. These people have (or had) tremendous energy or lived a very long time — or both! Some are extremists, some are more what you might think of as "balanced". It could be that some of the so-called extremists are really more in balance than any of us. Learn what they do and what they eat and how they live. Study health, not disease. Decide for yourself.

"Plant-based diets offer exceptional fuel for peak performance and optimal health at every stage of the life cycle. Organic vegetables, fruits, legumes, whole grains, nuts and seeds are loaded with vitamins, minerals, phytochemicals, antioxidants and fiber - the greatest protectors in the diet. They also effectively minimize the most damaging components in the diet - trans fatty acids, saturated fat, cholesterol, pro-oxidants, refined carbohydrates and environmental contaminants.

Plant-based diets are naturally high in the most healthful form of carbohydrates, helping athletes maximize glycogen stores, and allowing for harder work for longer periods of time. People choosing plant-based diets also reduce their lifetime risk of heart disease, cancer, type 2 diabetes, gastrointestinal diseases, gallbladder disease, and many immune/inflammatory disorders. While the advantages to our personal health are quite impressive, it is the advantages beyond our personal health that are perhaps most remarkable. Among the greatest contributions a person can make towards the preservation of this planet is eating simple, whole foods that are low on the food chain. Animal-centered, processed-food diets are not ecologically sustainable. Consuming a plant-based diet is also arguably the most powerful step a person can take to reduce cruelty, pain, suffering and death in this world. Plant-based diets are rooted in compassion and reverence for life."

—**Brenda Davis, R.D.**, author of ***Becoming Vegan*** and ***Becoming Vegetarian***.

"Every nutrient known to be essential for human health is available, in proper concentration, in plant foods. This is not so with animal-based foods, as there are many essential nutrients

totally absent in them. A diet consisting of whole fresh ripe raw organic plants is ideal for human health and performance as it most closely accommodates our anatomical and physiological needs for food. We are, literally, built to consume plants. In exactly the same fashion that a car will run best when supplied with the fuel for which it is designed, so too will humans be able to reach their fullest performance potential when utilizing the diet for which we are best built to accommodate."

— **Dr. Doug Graham**, author of ***Nutrition and Physical Performance***.

Rejuvelac Recipe from Ann Wigmore Institute, Puerto Rico

a. Soak. 2 cups soft wheat berries in purified water 8 hrs or overnight.
b. Drain, rinse, then allow to sprout for 2 days, without rinsing
c. When white sprout tails begin to show, add 6 cups purified water, cover jar with cheesecloth, put in a warm place where it can be exposed to at least 70 degree temp for 2 days.
d. THEN pour off, drink or refrigerate and use "Rejuvelac" in a raw blended soup recipe.
e. The leftover seeds can be used one more time, with 4 cups purified water, will culture in 1 day.
f. Then seeds can be composted, or thrown to birds.

MIKE'S THREE SIMPLE RULES FOR DIET SUCCESS

Eat at least 75% of your daily diet consisting of raw uncooked fruits and veggies. If you have a problem digesting any raw foods (that can normally be eaten that way by others and do not have to be cooked, such as artichokes or rhubarb), then use a VitaMix or similar blender to "chew" these highly digestible foods to a pulp, soup or puree and see how you "feel". Take 1-2 Ultimate Enzymes with EVERY meal and before bed. (http://www.healthnuts.net - use #2177 as your referral).

1. Add 2-4 tablespoons of freshly ground flax seeds per 16 ounces of fluid (http://www.dakotaflax.com) Also add Rejuvelac (see recipe above).
2. Do not consume any non-sprouted grains, fish or animal protein except salmon pasteurized dairy products,

chocolate, coffee, sugar, salt, spices except cayenne, fried foods, artificial colors.
3. Supplement all this with Optimal Breathing® Development. Make just those three changes and watch your lungs and overall health improve!

You'll LOVE Mike's daily smoothie: My daily smoothie consists of spinach, broccoli, one small apple, slice of fresh pineapple, flax seeds, safflower oil, olive oil, pomegranate or cranberry juice, alkaline water, almond milk, Sparx vitamin and mineral supplement, celery, zucchini, E3live flakes, spirulina, collard greens all in portions to taste. I vary them somewhat due to availability and freshness.

ALMOND MILK
Soak almonds for about 12 hours in pure water. You can also soak large amounts, rinse and drain and then put them in freezer bags in the freezer for later individual bag use).
1 cup soaked almonds
2 cups pure water
2 - 3 dates
1/4 tsp Celtic sea salt
Raw living foods containing simple carbohydrates. Minus their fiber content they are convertible into carbon dioxide. The fiber "brooms" the debris into the colon. Raw foods are the most enzyme laden and efficient processing of nutrients but not always the most practical. Fresh raw vegetable and fruit juices are concentrated with mega live nutrients, easiest to digest and are often extremely helpful for more challenging lung problems. Juicers abound. Juice feverishly — pun intended.

Individual health conditions and emergencies may require more creative approaches to optimal nutrition but gourmet raw foods can be a welcome addition to any palate and health program. Attend raw living foods potlucks to become more familiar with their variety, textures, tastes and
nutrition. Check out these websites: http://www.livingnutrition.com http://www.living-foods.com http://www.rawfood.com

Food Combining Chart
Doug Graham sells an easy one: *"Food Combining Simplified"* http://foodnsport.com/products/products.html

I'd start by keeping fruits separate from everything unless they are well Vita Mix blended with veggies. The blending "chews" foods and makes them much more digestible and more likely to be digested, even if you choose combinations that are not optimal. Eat starches separate from meats — always.

What's an Ideal Percentage Of Raw Foods?
If you're not eating 100% raw and have found your health does better with the addition of cooked foods, please join us for some great discussions at http://www.rawplus.com/community/

Your Natural Diet: Alive Raw Foods by Dr. T. C. Fry & David Klein is now available in paperback. (200 pages, $15.00 plus shipping). This book teaches the hygienic approach to healthful eating and lifestyle and it includes a full-page ad for **Healthful Living International**. It is the first new hygienic diet paperback printed since Dr. Shelton's books over 50 years ago! Contact publisher David Klein dave@livingnutrition.com or order online: http://www.livingnutrition.com/bookstore.html

Alkaline/Acid Balance
Acid/Alkaline balance is the "key" to health since the Standard American Diet (a.k.a. SAD) is mostly acid- forming foods.

ALKALINE FORMING FOODS

VEGETABLES
Alfalfa, Barley Grass, Asparagus, Fermented Veggies, Watercress, Beets, Broccoli, Brussels sprouts, Cabbage, Carrot, Cauliflower, Celery, Chard, Chlorella, Collard Greens, Cucumber, Eggplant, Kale, Kohlrabi, Lettuce, Mushrooms, Mustard Greens, Dulce, Dandelions, Edible Flowers, Onions, Parsnips (high glycemic), Peas, Peppers, Pumpkin, Rutabaga, Sprouts, Squashes, Wheat Grass, Wild Greens, sea weed, Blue green Algae such as E3live, spirulina, chl*orella and more sea weed

FRUITS
Apple, Apricot, Avocado, Banana (high glycemic), Cantaloupe, Cherries, Currants, Dates/Figs, Grapes, Grapefruit, Lime, Honeydew Melon, Nectarine, Orange, Lemon, Peach, Pear, Pineapple, All Berries, Tangerine, Tomato, Tropical Fruits, Watermelon

PROTEIN
Eggs (poached), Whey Protein Powder, Cottage Cheese, Chicken Breast, Yogurt, Almonds, Chestnuts, Tofu (fermented), Flax Seeds, Pumpkin Seeds, Tempeh (fermented), Squash Seeds, Sunflower Seeds, Millet, Sprouted Seeds, Nuts

OTHER
Apple Cider Vinegar, Bee Pollen, Lecithin Granules, Probiotic Cultures, Green Juices, Veggies Juices, Fresh Fruit Juice, Organic Milk, Mineral Water, Alkaline Antioxidant Water, Green Tea, Herbal Tea, Dandelion Tea, Ginseng Tea, Banchi Tea, Kombucha

SWEETENERS
Stevia, Ki Sweet

SPICES/SEASONINGS
Cinnamon, Curry, Ginger, Mustard, Chili Pepper, Sea Salt, Miso, Tamari, All Herbs

ORIENTAL VEGETABLES
Maitake, Daikon, Dandelion Root, Shitake, Kombu, Reishi, Nori, Umeboshi, Wakame, Sea Veggies

Extremely Alkaline Forming Foods - pH 8.5 to 9.0: Lemons, Watermelon , Agar Agar , Cantaloupe, Cayenne (Capsicum) , Dried dates & figs, Kelp, Karengo, Kudzu root, Limes, Mango, Melons, Papaya, Parsley , Seedless grapes (sweet), Watercress, Seaweeds

Moderate Alkaline - pH 7.5 to 8.0: Apples (sweet), Apricots, Alfalfa sprouts, Arrowroot, flour , Avocados, Bananas (ripe), Berries, Carrots, Celery, Currants, Dates & figs (fresh), Garlic , Gooseberry, Grapes (less sweet), Grapefruit, Guavas, Herbs (leafy green), Lettuce (leafy green), Nectarine, Peaches (sweet), Pears (less sweet), Peas (fresh sweet), Persimmon, Pumpkin (sweet), Sea salt (vegetable) , Spinach

Apples (sour), Bamboo shoots, Beans (fresh green), Beets, Bell Pepper, Broccoli, Cabbage; Cauliflower, Carob , Daikon, Ginger (fresh), Grapes (sour), Kale, Kohlrabi, Lettuce (pale green), Oranges, Parsnip, Peaches (less sweet), Peas (less sweet), Potatoes & skin, Pumpkin (less sweet), Raspberry, Sapote, Strawberry, Squash , Sweet corn (fresh), Tamari , Turnip, Vinegar (apple cider)

Slightly Alkaline to Neutral pH 7.0: Soaked almonds in water overnight, Artichokes (Jerusalem), Barley-Malt (sweetener-Bronner), Brown Rice Syrup, Brussels Sprouts, Cherries, Coconut (fresh), Cucumbers, Egg plant, Honey (raw), Leeks, Miso, Mushrooms, Okra, Olives ripe , Onions, Pickles (home made), Radish, Sea salt , Taro, Tomatoes (sweet), Vinegar (sweet brown rice), Water Chestnut, Amaranth, Artichoke (globe), Chestnuts (dry roasted), Egg yolks (soft cooked), Essene bread , Goat's milk and whey (raw) , Horseradish, Mayonnaise (home made), Millet, Olive oil, Quinoa, Rhubarb, Sesame seeds (whole)

, Soy beans (dry), Soy cheese, Soy milk, Sprouted grains, Tempeh, Tofu, Tomatoes (less sweet), Yeast (nutritional flakes)Soak the seeds and nuts and they become more alkaline.

ACTIVITIES THAT ARE MORE OFTEN ALKALINE THAN ACID FORMING:
Meditation, prayer, affirmations, relaxation, inner peace. sleep, peace, kindness, love, pleasant thoughts, smiles and optimal breathing.

ACID FORMING FOODS

FATS & OILS
Avocado Oil, Canola Oil, Corn Oil, Hemp Seed Oil, Flax Oil, Lard, Olive Oil, Safflower Oil,
Sesame Oil, Sunflower Oil

FRUITS
Cranberries

GRAINS
Rice Cakes, Wheat Cakes, Amaranth, Barley, Buckwheat, Corn, Oats (rolled), Quinoa,
Rice (all), Rye, Spelt, Kamut, Wheat, Hemp Seed Flour

DAIRY
Cheese (Cow), Cheese (Goat), Cheese (Processed), Cheese (Sheep), Milk, Butter

NUTS & BUTTERS
Cashews, Brazil Nuts, Peanuts, Peanut Butter, Pecans, Tahini, Walnuts

ANIMAL PROTEIN
Beef, Shellfish, Fish, Lamb, Lobster, Mussels, Oyster, Pork, Rabbit, Turkey, Venison.
Fish is easier to digest if it has trace minerals from its water environment.

PASTA (WHITE)
Noodles, Macaroni, Spaghetti

OTHER
Distilled Vinegar, Wheat Germ, Potatoes

BEANS & LEGUMES
Black Beans, Chick Peas, Green Peas, Kidney Beans, Lentils, Lima Beans, Pinto Beans, Red Beans,
Soy Beans, Soy Milk, White Beans, Rice Milk, Almond Milk

DRUGS & CHEMICALS
Aspartame, Artificial sweeteners, Chemicals, Drugs (Medicinal), Drugs (Psychedelic), Pesticides,
Herbicides

ALCOHOL
Beer, Spirits, Hard Liquor, Wine

ACID FORMING ACTIVITIES ARE:
Overwork, Anger, Fear, Jealousy, stress, poor sleep, over-training

** All foods head towards acidity when sugar is added or they are cooked, processed or refined **

** Rhubarb alkalizes but has properties bad for health.

BALANCE OF ACID ALKALINE
I believe that a good ratio of acid/alkaline foods would be 90% alkaline to 10% acid until vitality returns. A maintenance ratio would be 80% alkaline to 20% acid foods in the diet if a person is satisfactorily healthy.

FAT CELLS ARE A STORAGE SHED FOR ACID!

Our bodies produce fat to save our lives! The body creates fat cells to carry acids away from your vital organs, so these acids literally don't choke your organs to death. The American diet produces a lot of excess acid in our bodies. Acid tears down important body tissues, causing or worsening over 150 diseases, including the two big ones, heart disease and cancer.

Read Dr. Ted Baroody's book: ***ALKALIZE OR DIE***
THE pH MIRACLE by Dr. Robert Young has some valuable life-saving advice and recipes!

How do you know if you're overly acidic?

Parasites thrive on an acid base and do not want to be near oxygen, as it is like poison to them.

SPROUTS CAN SUPER CHARGE YOUR BODY!!
Germinating and sprouting are two simple processes of producing healthy and nutritious living foods. Germination is the soaking of seeds, nuts, beans and grains in water for a certain period of time. Sprouting is a continuation of germination, where the soaked seeds are grown for 2-5 days in glass jars, baskets or in a bed of soil.

<u>Sprouts</u> **are one of the most perfect foods because of their high levels of calcium and amino acids (building block of protein), vitamins and minerals, all in a highly digestive form. Pound per pound, sprouted beans and lentils contain as much protein as red meat - without the fat, cholesterol, hormones and antibiotics. They are also an excellent source of calcium!**

Cows, horses, pigs, gorillas, elephants, man and other animals eat GREENS every day –NOT meat! Human digestive tracts are made for greens, vegetables and fruits, seeds, sprouted grains and nuts! Dogs,cats,lions and other similar animals have short, highly acidic digestive tracts for digesting meat. Humans do NOT! Our intestines are over 22 ft. long.

Sprouts are packed with enzymes - the complex catalysts that initiate and control almost every chemical reaction in the human body. Sprouting is the most efficient way to use a whole food to its fullest benefits. It creates an enormous increase in the vitamin content of seeds — by several hundred percent with many vitamins! Various sprouted seeds, beans and grains contain abundant antioxidants, known to alleviate free radical damage.

The abundance of oxygen in these foods must not be ignored. On a living foods diet, a continual supply of oxygen is fed into your bodywith extremely beneficial results.

Sprout your own with equipment from. http://www.discountjuicers.com

http://www.RawFoodsNews.com
An online news magazine, featuring authoritative information, breaking news, and fun, interactive features on the raw vegan lifestyle. Rated Number 1 in the Webseed Directory's most interesting sites list, based on how many articles a person looks at in any one visit.

RAW RECIPE BOOKS
- The Sun food Diet Success System by David Wolfe
- Vibrant Living by Sally Pansing Kravich
- The Uncook Book by Elizabeth Baker
- Sweet Temptations by Frances Kendall
- Milk Recipes from Nuts & Seeds by Edith Edwards
- Soup Alive! By Eleanor Rosenast
- Dining in the Raw by Rita Romano & Nancy Jolly
- Hooked on Raw by Rhio
- Lover's Diet by Viktoras & Youkta Kulvinskas
- Raw Family by Victoria, Igor, Sergei &Valya Boutenko
- 12 Steps to Raw: Breaking The Cooked Foods Addiction by Victoria Boutenko

- The Raw Secrets by Frederic Patenaude
- The Raw Life by Paul Nison
- The High Energy Diet Recipe Guide by Douglas Graham
- Living in the Raw by Rose Lee Calabro
- Sproutman's Kitchen Garden Cookbook by Steve Meyerowitz
- Sunfood Cuisine by Frederic Patenaude
- Living Cuisine by Renee Loux Underkoffler
- Rainbow Green Live-Food Cuisine by Gabriel Cousens

Go to http://www.Fetchbook.info and punch in the name of the book you are looking for.... they will find the lowest price for you on any book.

TAKE COURSES ON A RAW FOOD LIFESTYLE

http://www.transformationinst.com/
http://www.healthfullivingintl.com/
http://www.tanglewoodwellnesscenter.com
http://www.foodnsport.com

FOOD ALLERGIES

"The most important action step you can take is to avoid food and food groups that cause allergic reactions."

Did you know that food allergies interfere with natural energy transmissions both in the brain and the body's cellular systems. People who have severe allergies tend to show a 2% to 3% decrease in arterial blood oxygen. Add that to a sick building's low oxygen environment, a rainstorm with another 5-10% less oxygen and you have less O_2 than is considered healthy.

Poor breathing causes excessive anxiety, which stimulates excessive adrenaline. To counter the high adrenaline the body produces histamine. This is why some people take anti histamine when they have a cold to reduce runny nose, sneezing and sinus blockage. Poor breathing also causes poor digestion that causes poor bowel function that causes backup of toxins that flood the lungs with excessive debris, which causes mucous production and copious free radicals.

To avoid allergic foods, learn terms used to describe these foods on foods labels, for example:
Milk protein - milk, non-fat milk solids, cheese, yogurt, and caseinates: whey, lactose.
Egg - eggs, egg albumen, egg yolk, egg lecithin
Lactose - milk, lactose.
Gluten - wheat, barley, rye, triticale, wheat bran, malt, oats, corn flour, oat bran
Soy - soybeans, hydrolysed vegetable protein, soy protein isolates, and soy lecithin.
Salicylates - strawberries and tomatoes.
A dietitian (or web search) can help you to learn to read food labels so you can avoid common allergens and allergic food.

<u>**Chocolate is a major allergen.**</u> Americans spend six billion dollars annually on chocolate. Why? Caffeine stimulates, fat satisfies and sugar entices and nurtures. The chocolate might not be so bad at the party if it didn't include other additives such as sugar — but try chocolate without sugar once to see how you like it. Many people eat chocolate when they start to feel negative or positive emotions. It is used as a mood altering substance then and is often triggered by an energetic/emotional issue that is being subdued. Immune system weakness also stems from this.
Drugs and many herbal tonics are potentially harmful as they stress and over stimulate the adrenal system without rebuilding. Give the body high energy producing natural food and it will not need or crave this. Breathe balanced and deeply and the nutrition will reach its full potential without being thrown off kilter by errant biochemical and emotional reactions.

Find some good books on allergies; there are dozens of them (suggestions in Appendix).

Allergic Reactions/Symptoms can include:
✘ Breathing difficulties, including wheezing and asthma
✘ Wheezing, any lung disorder
✘ Itching, burning and swelling around your mouth
✘ Nausea, vomiting, abdominal cramps and diarrhea
✘ Fatal anaphylaxis (the breathing tubes in your lungs tighten up and you can't breathe)
✘ Generalised urticaria - your skin becomes red and raised.

Four types of food allergy

Type I - Within 60 minutes of eating the food. The blood vessels dilate and the nose runs. This "ananaphylaxis" (hypersensitivity to proteins) can be life threatening.

Type II - causes similar symptoms to type I.

Type III - occurs some hours after eating and causes skin and bronchi (lung) irritation.

Type IV - is a delayed reaction that occurs 1-7 days after eating the food. Generally, the more of the food you eat, the worse your symptoms become.

Around 95 per cent of food allergies result in a Type IV reaction!

ASSESSING FOR FOOD ALLERGIES

Diet And Medical History

Factors in your diet and medical history that suggest food allergy include:
✘ Symptoms occur shortly after eating the food;
✘ Symptoms involve more than one body organ. (For example, swelling of the mouth and cramping of the abdomen);
✘ You have a family history of asthma, hay fever or dermatitis.

Diagnostic tests
The diagnostic tests used include:
✗ Skin and blood tests;
✗ Oral food challenges. Small doses of the food are given to you under   clinical conditions.
✗ Pulse rate. My favorite. Check pulse before eating food and if it   increases 10 beats per minute you are overly sensitive to that food.
✗ You cough up mucous after eating food you are overly sensitive to

See http://www.directlabs.com for an extensive list of very cost-effective laboratory fees that do not require a doctor's visit and the charges that go along with those tests.

CALCIUM FOR THE LUNGS – Be very careful where you get your calcium.

PLANTS ARE YOUR BEST SOURCE OF CALCIUM!

(and natural magnesium + instantly useable & highly-absorbable PROTEIN!)

From: Robert Cohen   http://www.notmilk.com

"Where do animals get their calcium? The answer is PLANTS (veggies) are loaded with calcium. Cows eat plants. Humans should too. Human breast milk is the perfect formula for baby humans. In her wisdom, Mother Nature included 33 milligrams of calcium in every 100 grams, or 3 1/2-ounce portion of human breast milk. At the end of this column are calcium values for 55 commonly eaten foods. Compare those calcium values to human breast milk.
    The perfect calcium-rich food is hummus. Chick Peas (150 mg) + sesame seeds (1160 mg) will yield a food containing ten

times as much calcium as human breast milk.

In order to absorb calcium, the body needs comparable amounts of another mineral element, magnesium. Magnesium is the center atom of chlorophyl. Milk and dairy products contain only small amounts of magnesium. Without the presence of magnesium, the body only absorbs 25 percent of the available dairy calcium content. The remainder of the calcium spells trouble. Without magnesium, excess calcium is utilized by the body in injurious ways. The body uses an unhealthy form of calcium to build the mortar on arterial walls that becomes atherosclerotic plaque (usually to fight excess acidity in the bloodstream)!

Excess calcium is converted by the kidneys into painful stones that grow in size like pearls in oysters, blocking our urinary tracts, kidneys, liver and gall bladder. Excess calcium contributes to arthritis. Painful calcium buildup often is manifested as gout.

Osteoporosis is NOT a problem that should be associated with lack of calcium intake. Osteoporosis results from calcium loss. The massive amounts of protein in milk result in a 50 percent loss of calcium in the urine. In other words, by doubling your protein intake there will be a loss of 1to 1.5 percent in skeletal mass per year in postmenopausal women.

"The calcium in leafy green vegetables is more easily absorbed than the calcium in milk
and plant proteins do not result in calcium loss the same way as do animal proteins."
—**Robert Cohen** http://www.notmilk.com

Calcium Content of Plants

01. Human Breast Milk 33 mg
02. **Almonds 234** mg
03. **Amaranth 267** mg
04. Apricots (dried) 67 mg
05. Artichokes 51 mg
06. Beans (can: pinto, black) 135 mg
07. Beet greens (cooked) 99 mg
08. Blackeye Peas 55 mg
09. Bran 70 mg
10. Broccoli (raw) 48 mg
11. Brussel Sprouts 36 mg
12. **Buckwheat 114** mg
13. Cabbage (raw) 49 mg
14. Carrot (raw) 37 mg
15. Cashew nuts 38 mg
16. Cauliflower (cooked) 42 mg
17. Swiss Chard (raw) 88 mg
18. **Chickpeas** (garbanzos) **150** mg
19. **Collards** (raw leaves) **250** mg
20. Cress (raw) 81 mg
21. **Dandelion** Greens **187** mg
22. Endive 81 mg
23. Escarole 81 mg
24. **Figs** (dried) **126** mg
25. **Filberts** (Hazelnuts) **209** mg
26. **Kale** (raw leaves) **249** mg
27. **Kale** (cooked leaves) **187** mg
28. Leeks 52 mg
29. Lettuce (lt. green) 35 mg
30. Lettuce (dark green) 68 mg
31. **Molasses** (dark-213 cal.) **684** mg
32. **Mustard Greens** (raw) **183** mg
33. **Mustard Greens** (cooked) **138** mg
34. Okra (raw or cooked) 92 mg
35. Olives 61 mg
36. Oranges (Florida) 43 mg
37. **Parsley 203** mg
38. **Peanuts** (roasted) **74** mg
39. Peas (boiled) 56 mg
40. **Pistachio Nuts 131** mg
41. Potato Chips 40 mg
42. Raisins 62 mg
43. Rhubarb (cooked) 78 mg
44. Sauerkraut 36 mg
45. **Sesame Seeds 1160** mg
46. Squash (Butternut) 40 mg
47. Soybeans 60 mg
48. Sugar (brown) 85 mg
49. **Tofu 128** mg
50. Spinach (raw) 93 mg
51. **Sunflower Seeds 120** mg
52. Sweet Potatoes (baked) 40 mg
53. Turnips (cooked) 35 mg
54. **Turnip Greens** (raw) **246** mg
55. **Turnip Greens** (boiled) **184** mg
56. **Water Cress 151** mg

Un-pasteurized milk drinkers beware. The cattle industry has tainted even the non-pasteurized source (with possibly the exception of organic beef) so it is risky to try non pasteurized milk — but it's still preferable to getting sick from pasteurized milk. Be careful and go raw as often as safe. Or do not drink milk at all.

Milk and Tuberculosis

According to Virgil Hulse, M.D. (author of Mad Cows and Milkgate), half of the dairy herds in America have cows testing positive for bovine tuberculosis. One cow infects another cow with tuberculosis. On January 10, 2005 America became aware of the Michigan hunter who caught bovine tuberculosis from a deer. The deer most likely ran out of the woods onto the cow's turf and became infected. This story should act as a warning to both hunter and dairy consumer.

Some say that half the dairy herds in America are infected with bovine tuberculosis. Others promote the consumption of raw milk. Neither thought should be comforting to milk and dairy consumers.

✗ "Infected raw milk is the chief means by which milk-borne tuberculosis is transmitted to man." — Journal of Dairy Science, 19:435, 1936.
✗ "Many diseases such as tuberculosis are transmissible by milk products." — **Journal of Dairy Science** 1988; 71
✗ "Some strains of mycobacteria, similar to those that are associated with tuberculosis, have been found to survive pasteurization." — **The National Mastitis Council, Inc.** 1970 Washington, D.C.

"A Mycobacterium bovis-infected dairy herd of 369 Holstein cows with lactation duration between 200 and 360 days was tested... 170 cows had positive tuberculin test results, and 199 had negative results."

 — *Journal of the American Veterinary Medical Association*, 1998 Sep, 213:6

MORE ABOUT MILK
http://www.notmilk.com
MILK from A to Z: http://www.notmilk.com/milkatoz.html
2O QUESTIONS: http://www.notmilk.com/notmilkfaq.html

As I said before everything works better when we integrate nutrition and breathing development. Begin with the **#176Video/ DVD** and **Diaphragm Strengthener**. (http://www.breathing.com/video-ds.htm)

FIBER HELPS CLEAN THE LUNGS AND KEEP THEM CLEAN
Fiber is the broom or shovel for your "intestinal debris".

FIBER AS AN ANTIOXIDANT?
Many studies focus on antioxidants. I think of fiber as a strong antioxidant, though it is not classified as such. If you had a 6-foot high pile of sticks and stones in your driveway and needed to remove them you would want a shovel and wheelbarrow. You would remove the large chunks of debris and then clean off the rest with a water hose. Trying to remove the 6-foot high pile with the water hose would be silly. That is what many try to do when they expect antioxidants to remove the debris that digestion and elimination has not.

Vegetables, fruits, whole grains and flaxseeds are good sources. Fiber is the broom that sweeps clean the cellular debris in the intestines, particularly the colon that otherwise collects and forms cellular debris, bacteria and phlegm.

A gentle intestinal cleansing and fiber source with almost every known fiber source on earth would be: Insulin Dietary Fiber: Oligo-fructose Dietary fiber (for stimulation of Bifidus), Apple Pectin, Guar Gum, Galascomannan fiber, Slippery elm, Cascara sagrada, Kelp, Charcoal powder, Chlorophyll, Zinc Gluconate, Chromium Nicotinate, Manganese Glycanate, copper, Potassium, Molybdenum aminochelate, iodine, Mucopolysaccharide, Aloe Vera Resin, Silymarin, Silica, Barley Grass powder, Arizona Barley Grass Juice Powder, Ride Bran, Butternut Bark, Plantain Ovata, Chaparral, Yellow Dock Root,

Rhubarb, Goldenseal root, Black cohosh, Triphala powder, marshmallow, licorice root powder. I've purposely omitted psyllium, as many are allergic to it.

Optional support includes using a Colema board, taking an enema, or monthly colonics and copious probiotics, including Threelac, to replenish the healthy bacteria lost due to excess water in the colon from the water cleansings.

From a raw food discussion group:
I suggest that you go to http://www.fitday.com and sign up for a free account. This will take you to a nutrition chart and database where you can input the food that you want to eat in a day. The database calculates the nutrition of the foods and gives you the calorie count and the percentages of carbs, fats, and protein. There is also a wheel that color codes these nutrients so that you get a very clear picture of what your daily diet would look like.

I did exactly this a few weeks ago when I was trying to work out a raw food diet that I could live with. I put in the food that I wanted to eat which was basically green veggie. I thought 2 cups per meal would be good, plus I cup other veggies like carrots and a few nuts for the essential fatty acids, plus the amount of fruit that I thought I would want to eat during the day around 2 to 3 items: apple and pears.

I was very surprised and pleased to see that I could eat just these foods and have an excellent balance of all the nutrients. I was particularly surprised to see how much protein there was. At lower calorie counts there was already 30% protein.

Proper diaphragm movement promotes intestinal cleansing!

The expansion and contraction of the diaphragm as it goes up and down causes movement. That movement translates into downward force to help the fiber be pushed out and the cellular debris along with it.

www.ama-assn.org/.../images/446/atlastorso.gif
American Medical Association website

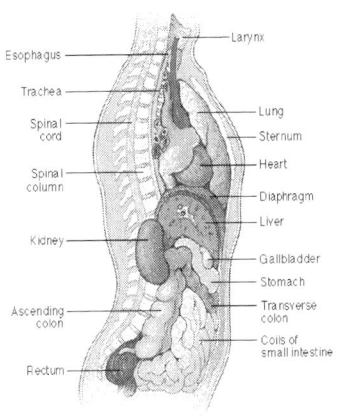

Body/Torso -- Side View

Your torso consists of two parts — the chest and the abdomen. The chest contains your heart and lungs; your abdomen contains the digestive and urinary systems. Your chest and abdomen are separated by a dome-shaped sheet of muscle called the diaphragm.

CHAPTER 7
Digestion and Elimination

The worse your digestion the more your breathing energy gets sidetracked to bear the burden of congestion and/or constipation. Poor digestion steals oxygen, diverts antioxidants and muddies up cellular function with cellular debris.

Digestion, just like breathing, in greater or lesser degree, must occur all the time to maintain optimum healthÉ not just in the stomach, upper and lower intestine and pancreas, but in the blood stream as well, and while you sleep.

Creating efficient digestion is as important as improving the way you breathe!

"Most people do not realize that conditions such as repetitive strain injuries, chronic fatigue syndrome, depression, energy swings, headaches, arthritis, fibromyalgia, depression, etc often have roots in one's digestive functioning." Dasha Trebichavska, L.AC.

The more cooked, canned and frozen foods you eat the more you need be concerned about digestion. Many allergies are caused by undigested foods in the blood stream. Undigested foods also cause both detected and hidden excessive mucous that clogs up the pathways of vital body fluids (blood, lymph, urine). This is just the *"tip of the iceberg"*. <u>**Poor breathing and poor digestion are factors in every chronic illness**</u>! When people drink liquids during meals, and take drugs that neutralize stomach acid, digestion becomes weak and incomplete. In-completely digested food creates toxins that interfere with the lymph and energy throughout the body. Acid reflux, hiatial hernia, irritable bowel syndrome, and Chron's Disease are a few *"symptoms"* of incomplete/poor digestion.

If the foods you eat are not completely digested, everything you do to try to establish (or maintain) optimal health will be considerably less effective!

Concernedabout weight control? Our all-natural enzyme combination lets you enjoy eating while you are losing weight. It processes your food so well that you eat less because your body is more efficiently breaking down what you eat, therefore getting more of the nutrition from your food. The enzymes pay for themselves by reducing your food consumption. Take 1-2 Ultimate Enzymes with EVERY meal and before bed.
(http://www.healthnuts.net -use #2177 as your referral)

A few more benefits of proper digestion and elimination.

- ✗ Take the load off your body and allow it to utilize its oxygen stores for recovery, regeneration and healing instead of processing food.
- ✗ Increase the surface area of your red blood cells... making it possible to carry more oxygen to all parts of your body
- ✗ Reduce or eliminate acid reflux
- ✗ Increase the white blood cell size and activity
- ✗ Breaking up cholesterol deposits
- ✗ Shatter crystalline deposits
- ✗ Stimulate the immune system
- ✗ Raise T-Cell activity and production
- ✗ Eliminate Yeast
- ✗ Reduce unhealthy bacteria
- ✗ Assimilate fats
- ✗ Digest proteins
- ✗ Offset lack of adequate chewing due to using dentures and partials.

TESTIMONIAL

"Hi Mike! You asked why I referred... My brother recently asked me how I lost 25 lbs I put him onto your site because I browsed "Optimal nutrition" and found the info about digestive enzymes from Optimal Digestion. I use them. They work!"

HOW MUCH ENZYMES IS ENOUGH?

How long do you want to live?

The father of modern day juicing, Norman Walker, lived to age 118.

According to Dr. Edwin Howell, the digestive system is designed to only break down approximately half of the food we eat. To appreciate a properly functioning digestive system, it helps to understand the 40 - 60 ratio theory discovered by Dr. Howell. Dr. Howell was one of America's pioneering biochemist and nutritional researchers and in his book ***"Enzyme Nutrition"*** he explains how the digestive system is designed to work. Before fire was discovered, man and animals alike could only eat raw food, like raw meat, plants or fruits and vegetables.

Raw foods have the 40 - 60 ratio, which means a raw food like an apple has live food enzymes within the apple that break down and digest 40 to 60 percent of that apple. This leaves the remaining 40 to 60% of the apple to be broken down by our digestive system.

There are only two types of food on earth: **1. Raw foods are enzymatically alive**, which means these foods have live enzymes within them to help digest 40 to 60% of that particular food. **2. Cooked and processed foods are enzymatically dead or denatured, which means there are NO live enzymes** within cooked foods to help digestion. These dead foods stress the digestive system, the pancreas, the immune system and much more.

I must bring this to your attention: almost all nutritional supplements are cooked and processed. If they don't have an excellent delivery system, there's a good chance you're not getting the benefits you thought you were giving your body.

Enzymes act like a natural magnet to attract fat, stimulate the body's natural metabolism, inhibit bad cholesterol and boost good cholesterol. They also aid tremendously in the process of weight loss and long-term weight management.

Back in the 1960s and earlier our raw foods contained the proper 40 -60 ratio. <u>Today our raw foods are genetically altered, mineral deficient and are being manipulated for longer shelf life, which means the raw food we eat today could be in a 20 - 80 ratio... which is asking the human body to digest and break down 80 % of that food.</u> This is an additional problem because we're already asking the human body to break down 100% of the cooked and processed foods and supplements we eat, and now, possibly 80% or more of the raw foods we eat. **We're really stressing the human body, every single day!**

   More about this via my online audio: http://www.breathing.com/video/introsite/9min.htm

COULD NOT CHEW IT BECAUSE IT WAS SO TOUGH?

Alligator meat is VERY tough and chewy. A friend emptied some of our Optimal Digestion capsules onto a small piece of cooked alligator. 20 minutes later she could cut the alligator piece with a fork.

   To the degree you are not eating 100% raw living foods and/or chew with removable teeth is the degree you need to supplement with digestive enzymes. Use our enzymes with hydrochloric acid in the day with meals and without hydrochloric acid at bedtime without food. **It doesn't matter what you eat if you do not digest it. Take 1-2 Ultimate Enzymes with EVERY meal and before bed.** (http://www.healthnuts.net -use #2177 as your referral)

SECRETS OF OPTIMAL DIGESTION BOOK
Down load our free *"Secrets of Optimal Digestion"* booklet for 100s of insights about how your health is effected and a simple common sense way to increase ease and dependability of weight control, energy increase, immune system strength, mental clarity and much, much more. 100's of reasons why taking the enzymes at bedtime gives you so much more benefit than just during the day. http://www.breathing.com/optimal-digestion.htm

The majority of colon cancers begin as benign polyps, which appear silently and often produce no symptoms except blood in the stool. Developing a regular screening regimen that includes testing for hidden blood in your stool (using a fecal occult blood test such as **LifeGuard®**), you can stop colorectal cancer before it has a chance to develop. For a more in-depth approach, order one or more of the vast array of discounted blood, urine stool tests at http://www.directlabs.com Intestinal products also available, such as for hyperpermeability (leaky gut) . http://www.directlabs.com/testtypes.php#DMSP

ELIMINATION
Exercise assists elimination. Moderate movement/exercise moves the lymph system and causes increased circulation and bowel activity.

Couch potatoes often collect massive amounts of impacted feces in the large intestine. This inhibits bowel function and backs up debris into the lungs.

The fiber (see chapter on Diet and Nutrition) from the fruits, seeds and veggies, plus adequate water, plus well digested foods (that do not overload the elimination system) allow for easy complete elimination of food based toxic waste.

Rebounding plus an oxygen concentrator are a great combination. http://www.breathing.com/programs.htm

Elimination may be safely accelerated with **OxyCleanse**. http://www.breathing.com/oxy-cleanse.htm It's not habit forming and helps oxygenate the intestinal tract and speeds digestion and elimination.

The skin is one of the primary organs of elimination. Far Infrared Saunas are also a wonderful adjunct to healthy elimination and detoxification. http://www.breathing.com/sauna.htm

The balanced expansion and contraction of the diaphragm creates parasympathetic enervation — this is the "rest and digest action" of the **Autonomic Nervous System**. Also, as your diaphragm goes up and down it causes downward movement. That movement translates into downward force to help the fiber be pushed out and the cellular debris along with it.

Unbalanced Dysfunctional Breathing (UDB) inhibits digestion and elimination.

The Autonomic Nervous System
(From *Health & Living* Magazine by Steve Nugent, NMD, PhD)

The somatic nervous system consists of nerves that convey messages from the sense organs to the central nervous system and then to the muscles and glands. The autonomic nervous system is a set of neurons controlling the heart, intestines and other organs.

The autonomic nervous system also has two parts — the **sympathetic** and **parasympathetic**. The sympathetic has two paired chains of ganglia (collections of neuron cell bodies). Axons extend from the sympathetic nervous system to the organs.

The sympathetic system increases heart and breathing rates and decreases digestive activity. Since all sympathetic ganglia are linked, they act together — "in sympathy" with one another.

The parasympathetic nervous system has functions related to, but generally opposite from, those of the sympathetic system. Although these systems oppose each other, they usually act simultaneously. However, the balance of activity may sometimes tilt more toward one system or the other, resulting in one side overtaking the other temporarily or continuously.

Parasympathetic activity decreases heart rate, increases digestive rate, and generally promotes energy-conserving, non-emergency functions. Energy conservation means slow fat burn but efficient fat storage, making consistently parasympathetic people more prone to weight problems... more than sympathetic people.

Affected by the <u>PARASYMPATHETIC</u> Nervous System:

- ✘ Brain (right)
- ✘ Hypothalamus (ant)
- ✘ Pituitary Gland (post.)
- ✘ Pineal Gland
- ✘ Parotid Gland
- ✘ Tonsils
- ✘ Thymus
- ✘✘ **LUNGS** ✘✘
- ✘ Liver
- ✘ Adrenal Cortex
- ✘ Stomach
- ✘ GallBladder
- ✘ Pancreas
- ✘ Spleen
- ✘ Duodenum
- ✘ Intestines (L & S)
- ✘ Appendix
- ✘ Bone Marrow
- ✘ Immune System
- ✘ Lymphatic System
- ✘ Metabolism

Affected by the <u>SYMPATHETIC</u> Nervous System:

- ✘ Brain (left)
- ✘ Thalamus
- ✘ Hypothalamus (post.)
- ✘ Pituitary Gland (ant.)
- ✘ Parathyroid
- ✘ Thyroid
- ✘ Heart
- ✘ Adrenal Medulla
- ✘ Kidneys
- ✘ Ureter
- ✘ Prostate
- ✘ Bladder
- ✘ Ovaries
- ✘ Uterus
- ✘ Urethra
- ✘ Testes

CHAPTER 8.
Water

Unless you have bad kidneys, begin the day with two 8 oz glasses of water as soon as you get out of bed. You lose that much during sleep!

Dr. F. Batmanghelidj author of *"Your Body's Many Cries for Water"* recommends this in his books and at http://www.watercure.com and I highly support the increased addition of water to your morning and daily routine! As we age we dehydrate and lose our sense of thirst. This water in the early A.M. will help to get your body used to more water and this also helps to rehabilitate your thirst cravings — worked for me! You can get a lot more information about water at the http://www.watercure.com web site. Start with one ounce of water for every 2 pounds of body weight per day. Raw food advocates say water in fruits can count a great deal but read Dr. B's books to get the most accurate information, then decide for yourself.

Consider getting a water alkalizer http://www.breathing.com/warter-alkalizer.htm

"Human cells are mostly water and the human body is roughly 60% water by weight."
— (Gerstein M, and Levitt M, Scientific American, November 1998).

To put the above information into perspective, consider the words written by Sir Robert McCarrison, Director of the Laboratory of Human Nutrition, University of Oxford, in the Cantor Lectures to the Royal Society in 1936:

"Strictly speaking, BOTH oxygen and water are to be treated as foods, for of all the supplies on which the body are dependent, they are chief."
— McCarrison, R., Nutrition and Health, 1961.

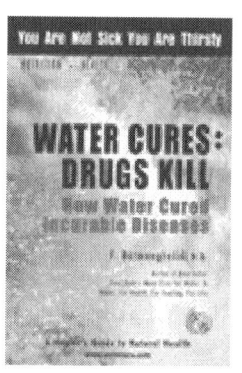

YOU'RE NOT SICK — YOU'RE THIRSTY!

Why 94 diseases get cured naturally with water!
by F. Batmanghelidj, M.D. • http://www.watercure.com

Sorry to report that Dr. Batman died in Nov. 2004. He was a hard working and dedicated health professional but he, as many of us do, had somewhat of a blind side. He had asthma. Mike invited him to develop his breathing. He lived a half days drive from Mike. He never showed up. He died of pneumonia.

"Dr. Batman" (as he liked to be called) left us vital data related to water. Nothing quenches your thirst like good old-fashioned H_2O, and it helps you lose weight, too. Drink at least 8—12 glasses a day. I suggest alkalized water using an alkalizer. http://www.breathing.com/water/alkalizer.htm Keeping water in plastic containers for too long, or reusing them can result in the plastic leaching into the water.

While reading another of Dr. Batman's books, **WATER CURES: DRUGS KILL**, you will learn that the medical industry has been defrauding society by forcing the use of toxic chemical medications when <u>the body is only manifesting signs of deep dehydration.</u> It's now clear that the pharmaceutical industry has invented most of our modern diseases — more than 94 of them!! Discover what these diseases are and how easily water can reduce or eliminate them. Learn his perspective about how allergies, asthma, hypertension, constipation and diabetes are caused or worsened by poor water management. **Discover why different pains in the body are actually indicators of what he called "regional drought" and we call --thirst.** Discover why cancer is caused by persistent dehydration in the fourth dimension of TIME.

More About Water

Dry mouth is not a reliable indicator of thirst because the body produces ample saliva. Producing saliva even in a dehydrated state is an over-riding primary function in the body to facilitate the act of chewing and swallowing food. Over salivation begins when the body is short of sodium (sea salt is best), a component of dehydration.

Hydrolytic actions of water drive all chemical reactions in our bodies. Histamine is a neurotransmitter in the body and is primarily a water regulator before its other functions. Chronic dehydration is a primary cause of pain and disease in the human body. Water is a primary inflammation-reducing remedy that helps prevent diseases associated with inflammation.

The following information comes from the book,
"Water...for health, for healing, for life" by F. Batmanghelidj, M.D.
- ✘ Without water nothing lives
- ✘ Water is the main source of energy - it is the "cash flow" of the body
- ✘ Water generates electricity and magnetic energy inside each and every cell of the body - it provides the power to live.
- ✘ Water prevents DNA damage and makes its repair mechanism more efficient.
- ✘ Water is used to transport all substances inside the body.
- ✘ Water increase the efficiency of red blood cells in collecting oxygen in the lungs. When water reaches the cell, it brings the cell oxygen and takes the waste gases to the lungs for disposal.
- ✘ Water clears toxic waste from the different parts of the body and takes it to the liver and kidneys for disposal.
- ✘ Water is the main lubricant in joint spaces.
- ✘ Water gives us power and electrical energy for all brain functions, most particularly thinking

Vocal Cords and Water

When vocal cords are not properly lubricated with phlegm (mucous), they redden and swell. This forms callus-like hard masses called nodules that keep the vocal cords from fully closing. I've read they can still cause problems after being surgically removed. To stay out of vocal trouble you need to remove any strain from your voice. If you are considering surgery , PLEASE consider first developing your breathing and voice with one of our **OBDSPAs** (Optimal Breathing Development Singing, Speaking and Personal Power specialists). http://www.breathing.com/school/results.htm or htm http://www.breathing.com/school/refer/main.htm

To make reasonably sure you are drinking enough water watch the color of your urine. Any color indicates you need more water (taking B vitamins and some medicines color your urine yellow or cause it to be unclear).

The water you drink should be room or body temperature, because water that is too cold constricts and water that is too hot over dilates the mucous membranes. **It takes extra ENERGY for your body to cool or heat that water.** That's why you should drink water in the first place- for more energy!

Vocal wise, diuretics such as caffeine, wine, tea, or soda cause your mucous to get more concentrated, causing excessive throat clearing. Sugar and acid-forming foods such as dairy and alcohol also cause thickening of mucous.

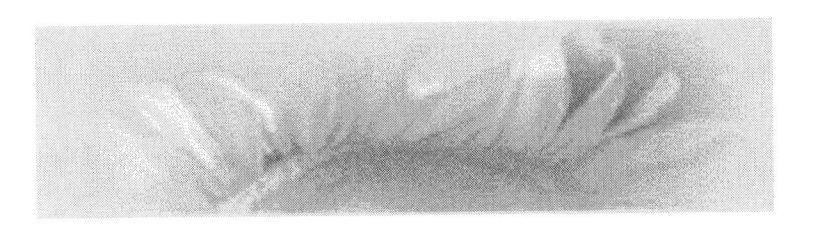

CHAPTER 9
THE IMPORTANCE OF SUNSHINE and SUNLIGHT

Are You Getting Enough Outdoor Light?
Our natural body rhythms are synchronized by the changing light of the sun from dawn to dusk. We need at least twenty minutes of natural light every day to keep our natural rhythms in working order.

Unfortunately, for our health, very few people get more than a few minutes of outdoor light (unimpeded by windows and glasses) in the winter months. This leads to SAD (Seasonal Affective Disorder).

Do you exhibit "symptoms" of sunlight deficiency?

- ✗ Does your full body skin receive fifteen to twenty minutes of full-spectrum light without sunscreen every day?
- ✗ Do you suffer from any sleep disorders?
- ✗ If you don't get 20 minutes of natural light a day, do you supplement vitamin D?
- ✗ Do you wear UV – blocking sunglasses?
- ✗ Do you believe that bright light is bad for you?
- ✗ If you are elderly you need five times more natural light to regulate the Circadian Rhythm than younger people. Do you receive enough?
- ✗ Do you have Seasonal Affective Disorder?
- ✗ Do you feel stress?

✗ Do you get sick frequently?
✗ Is your cholesterol high?
✗ Do you have psoriasis?
✗ Is your sex drive low?

Any of the above could mean that more sunshine is needed.

Forty percent of the population is considered deficient in Vitamin D!

Our bodies (most importantly our eyes), need fifteen to twenty minutes of exposure to the full-spectrum sunlight without sunscreens or UV blocking glasses every day in order for the skin to manufacture vitamin D.

Overuse of UVB sunscreen can interfere with vitamin D manufacture. Eyeglasses and windows also interfere with absorbing full-spectrum sunlight.

The light brightness measurement is called a **lux**. For therapeutic reasons you need to be exposed to light that is at least as bright as dawn or twilight, of 2,500 – 10,000 lux — even on cloudy days. Regular incandescent light bulbs don't even get close, producing 500-1,000 lux on the work surface. If you think that so-called full spectrum lighting is as good as sunlight, try reading a book in the sunshine and then in "full spectrum" light and "see" for yourself which works better.

When natural light is absorbed by the retina of the eye, electrical impulses are carried along the optic nerve to the brain and the hypothalamus, pineal gland, and pituitary gland, where it is used by the body to activate neurotransmitters that turn on many hormonal systems, including the metabolism, reproductive functions, and the internal biological clock called the **Circadian Rhythm**.

The Circadian Rhythm of the body is activated by light that is significantly brighter and more complex in spectrum than that which is needed for visual work. NASA installs full-spectrum lighting in spacecraft for this reason. It helps.

Light exposure raises <u>seratonin</u>, which <u>keeps you awake and alert.</u>
Melatonin rises in the dark, which makes you sleepy. It is suppressed by daylight. If you don't get enough light of sufficient intensity (lux) you produce too much melatonin, which makes you groggy. (If you are tired during the day, you might go out and get some sun!)
   Too much of a good thing can become a bad thing. Ionizing radiation creates free radicals that damage cells and are associated with cancer. Diet (antioxidants) and lifestyle factors can remove the free radicals and accelerate the repair of any damage they have caused. The ultraviolet rays that cause sunburn also produce vitamin D that is necessary for calcium absorption and may aid cancer prevention. Just be moderate with your sun exposure and you will reap MANY health benefits!

ACTION STEPS
Bathe your eyes in natural outdoor light without any glasses for up to 20 minutes every day. Soak it up - in a walk, on a deck, in a lawn chair, at the beach. Through your eyes, light goes directly to the hypothalamus, and from there to every cell in your body and it helps your skin manufacture Vitamin D, an essential nutrient. Work with a natural Vision trainer such as http://www.visionsofjoy.org I know Joy personally and you will get the very BEST attention.
   Take your lunch break outdoors whenever you can. You don't need to be in the direct sun. A porch is fine!
   Take the opportunity to read the daily newspaper in the sun; look at your mail there, too. In the winter, walk somewhere that isn't icy, so that you stay warm.
   If you are disabled, infirm, or unable to get outside for whatever reason, including living in a city, sit by an open window for 20 minutes or so every day, if it isn't too cold.

Sleep Deprived Baby?
Try Sunlight http://www.mercola.com/2004/dec/8/baby_sleepin.htm If you are having a hard time getting your baby to sleep through the night, you might want to consider a natural

solution: SUNLIGHT. Find out why exposure to light plays a crucial role in your infant's sleep behaviors and learn how to reap the benefits of sunlight during the cold winter months.

With proper diet and supplementation (see your health ND and/or professional about this) everyone, including cancer patients, can increase their tolerance for sunlight, thereby enjoying more health benefits that sunlight can provide by intake of appropriate nutrients. The impact of sunlight on the skin will become more controversial as the years go by. This is partly due to continued pollution-caused destruction of the earth's ozone layer that blocks UV radiation.

SUNBATHING HELPS HEAL ALMOST EVERYTHING!
Heliotherapy - the practice of sunbathing (search engine it)

Dr. Zane R. Kime writes *"those who get more sunlight have less cancer. Sunbathing heals cancer by building up the immune system and increasing the oxygen in the tissues. Sunlight does not cause skin cancer. Healthy people do not get cancer and - unhealthy people do get it. Chronic sunburn combines with free radicals to cause skin cancer. Sunlight may change free radicals, dietary fat, cholesterol and deranged antioxidants via cooked foods into skin cancer. Under the influence of sunlight, these toxic foods are brought to the skin. Cooked foods have had their antioxidants, particularly vitamins C and E, reduced or deranged by cooking. The sources of free radicals are mainly dietary fat, especially polyunsaturated fats, but also fats and oils applied to the skin in suntan lotion and other cosmetics. Suppression of the 'immune system by drugs may be involved in skin cancer that is stimulated by sunlight. X-rays and chemotherapy cause cancer."*

According studies documented by: Dr. Z. Kime, Sunlight, World Health Publications)
✠ Exposure to sunlight increases the body's ability to metabolize cholesterol, leading to a 13% decrease in blood cholesterol levels. (New England Journal of Medicine)

✠ *Studies indicate that exposure to UV light may have similar effects as exercise: a decrease in blood pressure, a lower resting heart rate, and a 39% increase in the heart's output of blood. (University of Frankfurt, Germany)*
✠ *Reports from the National Psoriasis Foundation indicate that 80% of those suffering from this skin disease improve when they are exposed to UV light.*

✠ *Sunlight and UV exposure may aid in the prevention of the common cold. Ten minutes of exposure to UV light one to three times a week has been demonstrated to reduce the frequency of colds up to 40.3%. Another study conducted with 4,000 male college students showed a link between more sunlight exposure and fewer colds. (Dr. Z. Kime, Sunlight, World Health Publications)*

Great information about sun gazing. A little extreme but with deep truths to offer. Decide for yourself. http://www.sungazing.com

I have a neighbor who is 66 and has emphysema, skinny as a rail, eats junk food and smokes like a chimney. I wondered what is keeping her alive and then recalled that she sunbathes almost every day. Hmmmmm..

I also used the strapping technique on her that is taught in the **#176 DVD/video** Fundamentals of Optimal Breathing® Program: http://www.breathing.com/video-strap.htm

CHAPTER 10
Nutritional Supplementation

Optimal nutrition classifies the degenerative diseases as deficiency disorders that should be prevented by proper water and nutrition — not by chemical drugs!
  I believe that supplementation is absolutely necessary. See your health professional or the product label for proper quantities. Be very cautious about anecdotal health benefit sharing of friends selling multilevel products. Many are valuable— but are they for YOU?

Note from Jan Jenson: *"Learn kinesiology (muscle testing), dowsing and/or how to use a pendulum and take charge of your own health needs. Your body (your higher self) will help you choose what is right for you!"*

Many people believe that eating a well balanced diet provides all the vitamins and minerals necessary for good health. In ideal circumstances, this is the case, but in reality there are many reasons why you may need vitamin supplements to cope with living in the twentieth century environment. Taking vitamins when required is a safe method of optimizing your dietary sources of nutrients, providing you follow the instructions of your health professional.
  Remember that dietary shortfalls can actually hinder brain function and sound reason. Don't be like the man who represents himself in court and have a fool for a client.

24 Reasons To Take Vitamin Supplements

This collection is not even close to complete and is offered to stimulate your curiosity to learn more about your specific needs:.

1. Poor Digestion
Even when your food intake is good, inefficient digest-ion can limit your body's uptake of vitamins, minerals, trace minerals and essential fatty acids. Some common causes of inefficient digestion are not chewing well enough due to too few chomps and chews or dentures (did you know that removable dentures are up to 85% less efficient in chewing than your own real teeth) and eating too fast, which results in larger-than-normal food particle size, which invites food allergy and constipation. Also, food particles that are too large will inhibit complete action of digestive enzymes.

2. Hot Coffee, Tea and Spices
Liquids consumed with meals dilute your digestive juices. Frequent drinking of liquids that are too hot, or con-suming an excess of irritants such as coffee, tea or pickles and spices can cause inflammation of the digestive linings, resulting in a reduction of secretion of digestive fluids and poor extraction of vitamins and minerals from food.

3. Alcohol
Excessive alcohol consumption is known to damage the liver and pancreas, which are vital to digestion and metabolism. It can also damage the lining of the intestinal tract and adversely affect the absorption of nutrients, leading to sub-clinical malnutrition. Regular heavy use of alcohol increases the body's need for the B-group vitamins, particularly thiamine, niacin, pyridoxine, folic acid and vitamins B, A and C as well as the minerals zinc, magnesium and calcium. Alcohol inhibits availability, absorption and metabo-lism of nutrients.

4. Smoking
Smoking 'too much tobacco' is also an irritant to the digestive tract and increases the metabolic require-ments of Vitamin C, all else being equal, by at least 30 mg per cigarette over and above the typical requirements of a non-smoker. Vitamin C, which is normally present in such fruits, will oxidize rapidly once these fruits are cut, juiced, cooked or stored in direct light or near heat. Vitamin C is very important to immune function.

5. Laxatives
Overuse of herbal laxatives can result in poor absorption of vitamins and minerals from food, by hastening the intestinal transit time. Some mineral oils increase losses of fat-soluble vitamins A, E and K. Other laxatives used to excess can cause large losses minerals such as potassium, sodium and magnesium.

6. Fad Diets
Bizarre diets that miss out on whole groups of foods can be seriously lacking in vitamins. Even the popular low fat diets, if taken to an extreme, can be deficient in vitamins A, D and E. Vegetarian diets, which exclude meat and other animal sources, must be very skillfully planned to avoid vitamin BI2 deficiency, which may lead to anemia.

7. Overcooking
Lengthy cooking or even worse, reheating of meat (possibly spoiled or rancid) and vegetables can oxidize and destroy heat susceptible vitamins such as the B-group, C and E. Boiling vegetables leaches the water soluble vitamins B-group and C as well as many minerals. Preferably raw or sometimes light steaming is preferable. Some vitamins, such as vitamin B6 can be destroyed by irradiation from microwaves.

8. Food Processing
Freezing food containing vitamin E can significantly reduce its levels. Foods containing vitamin E exposed to heat and air can turn rancid. Many common sources of vitamin E, such as bread and oils are nowadays highly processed and reduces or destroys

all vitamin E . Any process that increases storage life will probably lower nutrient levels. Vitamin E is an antioxidant, which defensively inhibits oxidative damage to all tissues. Other vitamin losses from food processing include vitamin B. and C.

9. Convenience Foods
A diet overly dependent on highly refined carbo-hydrates, such as sugar, white flour and white rice, places greater demand on additional sources of B -group vitamins to process these carbohydrates. An unbalanced diet contributes to such conditions as irritability, lethargy and sleep disorders.

10. Antibiotics
Some antibiotics (although valuable in fighting infect-ion) also kill off friendly bacteria in the gut, which would normally be producing B-group vitamins to be absorbed through the intestinal walls. Such deficiencies can result in a variety of nervous conditions. Therefore, it may be advisable to supple-ment with B-group vitamins and especially probiotics when on a lengthy course of broad-spectrum antibiotics.

11. Food Allergies
The omission of whole food groups from the diet as in the case of individuals allergic to gluten or lactose can mean the loss of significant dietary sources of nutrients such as thiamine, riboflavin or calcium.

12. Crop Nutrient Losses
Most agricultural soils are deficient in trace minerals (and have been since the 1930's!). Decades of intensive agriculture can overwork and deplete soils unless all the soil nutrients, including trace elements, are regularly replaced. This means that food crops can be depleted of nutrients due to poor soil management. In one U.S. Government survey, levels of essential minerals in crops were found to have declined by up to 68 per cent over a four-year period in the 1970's. In 2004-2005 it is doubtful that trend has improved.

13. Accidents & Illness
Burns lead to a loss of protein and essential trace nutrients such as vitamins and minerals. Surgery increases the need for zinc, vitamin E and other nutrients involved in the cellular repair mechanism. The repair of broken bones will be retarded by an inadequate supply of calcium and 'vitamin C and conversely enhanced by a full dietary supply. The challenge of infection places high demand on the nutritional resources of zinc, magnesium and vitamins B5, B6 and zinc.

14. Stress
Chemical, physical and emotional stresses can increase the body's requirements for vitamins B2, B5. B6, B12 and C. Air pollution increases the requirements for vitamin E.

15. P.M.T. & P.M.S.
Research has demonstrated that up to 60 per cent of women suffering from symptoms of pre-menstrual tension, such as headaches, irritability, bloatedness, breast tenderness, lethargy and depression can benefit from supplementation with vitamin B6.

16. Teenagers.
Rapid growth spurts, such as in the teenage years, place high demands on nutritional resources to underwrite the accelerated physical, biochemical and emotional development in this age group.

17. Pregnant Women
Pregnancy creates higher than average demands for nutrients to ensure healthy growth of the baby and comfortable confinement for the mother. Nutrients that typically need to be increased during pregnancy are the B-group, especially B1, B2, B3, B6 folic acid and B12, A, D, E and the minerals calcium, iron magnesium, zinc and phosphorous.

18. Oral Contraceptives
Oral contraceptives can decrease absorption of folic acid and increase the need for vitamin B6 and possibly vitamin C, zinc and riboflavin.

19. Light Eaters
Some people eat very sparingly, even without weight reduction. Under eating can cause deficiencies in thiamine, calcium and iron.

20. The Elderly
The elderly have been shown to have a low intake of vitamins and minerals, particularly iron. calcium and zinc. Essential fatty acid and folic acid deficiency is often found in conjunction with vitamin C deficiency. Fiber intake is often low. Riboflavin (B2) and pyridoxine (B6) deficiencies have also been observed. Possible causes include impaired sense of taste and smell. Reduced secretion of digestive enzymes, chronic disease and sometimes physical impairment.

21. Lack of Sunlight
Invalids, shift workers and people whose exposure to sunlight may be minimal can suffer from insufficient amounts of vitamin D which is required for calcium metabolism, without which rickets and osteoporosis (bone thinning) has been observed. Ultraviolet light is the stimulus to vitamin D formation in skin. It is blocked by cloud, fog, smog, smoke and ordinary window curtains and clothing.

22. Bio-Individuality
Wide fluctuations in individual nutrient requirements from the official recommended average vitamin and mineral intakes arc common, particularly for those in high physical demand vocations, such as athletics and manual labor. Taking into account body weight and physical type, protein intake influences the need for vitamin B6 and for some proteins can be satisfied with fresh fruits and vegetables.

23. Low Body Reserves
Although the body is able to store reserves of certain vitamins such as A and E, Canadian autopsy data bas shown that up to thirty percent of the population have reserves of vitamin A so low as to be judged "at risk". Vitamin A is important to healthy skin and mucous membranes (including the sinus and lungs) and eyesight.

24. Athletes

Athletes consume large amounts of food and experience considerable stress. These factors affect their needs for B-group vitamins, vitamin C and iron in particular. Tests on many athletes, such as football players, have shown wide ranging vitamin deficiencies.

The depth to which breathing obstructions go are not just limited to the lungs. The sinuses are a primary player. Most people don't realize that the sinuses are huge and go way back into the head.

Mike's Note: I bolded the products I personally would start with for lung health but you should consult a health professional for the exact balance of all this.

MAIN THEME.
Lungs, sinus, digestion, cleansing, detoxification, anti-fungal

1. *Acetyl-L-carnitine*
2. Alpha-lipoic acid,
3. **Beta Carotene**
4. Biotin. A B-Vitamin, helpful for lung conditions.
5. Boron. Used for infections. Very good for the lungs.
6. Bronchial Tissue Extract supports & strengthens the bronchials. Important be-cause it targets the bronchial tree
7. Cordyceps – Herbal combination – good for allergies. http://www.breathing.com/programs.htm
8. **Caprilic acid — oregano** (an herb) excellent for bronchial problems.
9. **Coenzyme Q10 — an oxygen-producing coenzyme for the body.**
10. Colloidal Silica — **supports the lung alveoli.**
11. **Colloidal Silver – natural antibiotic**
12. Coltsfoot. Used for centuries as a cough dispeller by ancient heal-ers such as Dioscorides, Galen & Pliny.

13. Columbine Flowers. A St. Hildegard favorite for infections of the rows of lymph glands in the neck, particularly in children. Good for sinusitis
14. Comfrey Root - good for the lungs, especially for coughing
15. DMG. Another oxygen-producing substance. Helps brain oxy-gen levels.
16. DMSO. Strong oxygen transport.
17. **Echinacea.** Excellent for viruses and bacterium.
18. **Fiber - 30-50 grams daily** light brown flax seeds from Dakota Flax grind fresh in a dedicated coffee grinder. http://www.dakotaflax.com
19. From Dr. James Biddle. For pulmonary fibrosis, add melatonin 6-18 mg at bed. Plus Zinc lozenges 80 milligrams total including all other supplements
20. **Garlic** natural or (Kyolic) protects against pneumonia.
21. **Germanium Sequioxide.** In supplements or in E3Live: http://www.breathing.com/e3live.htm **Green foods *You're My Everything*** from E3Live http://www.breathing.com/e3live.htm contains spirulina, chlorella, MSM and others.
22. **Ginger**
23. **Goldenseal**
24. **Glutathione.** August 2002 issue of ***Nutrition & Healing*** newsletter, Jonathan V. Wright, M.D., discusses COPD at length, and states that *"nebulized, inhaled glutathione is the No. 1 natural treatment for COPD in my practice."* Regular e-Alert readers will recognize glutathione as the powerful antioxidant and amino acid molecule.
25. **Histidine.** An amino acid used for its antihistaminic abilities.
26. Horseradish — table spoon with lemon juice for phlegm
27. **Juice carrots, spinach** - see Norman Walker's Fresh Vegetable Juices book
28. Kelp
29. **Lipoic acid**
30. **Lungwort.** favorite of S1 Hildegard of Bingen for all lung problems.
31. **Magnesium.**
32. Mullein. can stop bleeding in the lungs and create an overall strengthening

33. **Olive Leaf Extract**
34. **Oregano oil,** VERY potent bug killer for the lungs http://www.breathing.com/oregano-oil.htm
35. Pleurisy Root. Used by ancient healers to help pleurisy.
36. **Probiotics** — ProFlora - purchase at http://www.breathing.com/programs.htm
37. **ProEfa** - Essential fatty acids. Fish oil, borage etc. breathing.com programs page
38. **Protease, Amylase, Lipase, Bromelain.** Used to assist the digestion of protein, fat & carbohydrates. See http://www.breathing.com/optimal-digestion.htm
39. **Pycnogenol**. Major antioxidant
40. **Quercetin**. Antioxident/bioflavonoid used for its anti-histamine properties to assist the sinuses.
41. **Sandalwood** (Santalum Album) lungs & sinuses. Used for 2000 years with great success in the Tibetan medical tradition
42. Selenium
43. **Taurine**
44. **Thyme.** Culpepper, stated that Thyme is "a noble strengthener of the lungs."
45. **Umeboshi Plum.** Alkalizing properties to lungs & sinuses.
46. **Vitamin A emulsion** — vitamin A precautions. Beta carotene is the precursor to vitamin A. Use carrot juice as the source or encapsulated supplementation
47. **Vitamin B2** (riboflavin) Helps mild asthma if taken consistently..
48. **Vitamin C** daily to bowel tolerance –
49. **Vitamin E**
50. **Water** http://www.breathing.com/articles/water-doc.htm
51. **Oxywater** http://www.breathing.com/oxywater.com
52. We need oxygen and we need water. The best of BOTH worlds from http://www.Oxywater.com
53. **Wheat Gras**s Fresh 1 oz 2 times daily
54. **Yakriton.** A liver extract that is a very good anti-histamine.
55. Food-allergy rotation diets, magnesium, and vitamins B-6, B-12, and C are a popular combination.

Antifungal
Clarkia. DOUBLE Tincture – Extra Strong
Proflora - oodles of it http://www.breathing.com/proflora.htm
Threelac
Caprilic acid

Cleansing
Oxycleanse. Gentle, non-habit forming. Ok for long-term use: http://www.breathing.com/oxy-cleanse.htm
Arise and Shine – Cleanse and Heal Thyself. One of the best. http://www.ariseandshine.com
Jon Cotton's great program at http://www.Totalhealthsecrets.com

Books etc
Norman Walker's **Fresh Vegetable Juices**. Easy on the sweet ones due to candida and diabetes.
Juicers from http://www.discountjuicers.com
Any book by Paul Bragg

Subscribe to *Living Nutrition Magazine* at http://www.livingnutrition.com

Multi Vitamin Supplements
Over 5,000 supplements from TID Health http://www.tidhealth.com
Immune Support — http://www.breathing.com/immune.htm
SPARX — purchase at http://www.breathing.com/sparx.htm

Homeopathy. Can be very helpful. http://www.breathing.com/programs.htm
Look for King Bio products

REGENERATING ALVEOLI with nutrition — instead of drugs !
Scientists funded by the **National Heart, Lung and Blood Institute** have demonstrated a remarkable regeneration of alveoli, which returned to their normal size and number.

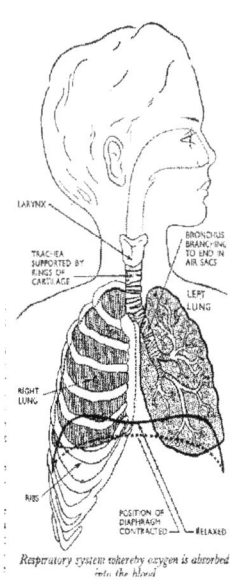

In research using rats at the Georgetown University School of Medicine, treatment with **retinoic acid, a metabolite of vitamin A,** resulted in a non-surgical reversal of damage caused by emphysema for the first time. Not only was the number of alveoli increased in normal rats, but alveoli in rats with emphysema were repaired and lung elasticity recoil was significantly improved. Though these studies have so far been conducted only in animals, results are very promising, leading a number of physicians to put their emphysema patients on retinoic acid therapy.

Respiratory system whereby oxygen is absorbed into the blood

This points to why many people live quite well following strict nutritional guidelines and moderate exercise.

I am hopeful that this remarkable nutritional-based therapy will be more widely adopted. In fact, the FDA may be approving all-trans-retinoic acid for emphysema therapy. All-trans-retinoic acid must now be prescribed by a physician.

To accelerate success with this process I highly recommend you integrate the techniques in our Breathing **#176** Development Fundamentals program http://www.breathing.com/video-strap.htm

Chapter 11
Hair, Urine, Fecal, Lung and Blood Testing

Hair analysis
Hair mineral analysis offers you a clear understanding of your body's mineral and trace element levels. It can usually identify inorganic toxic materials that may be present so that appropriate treatments can be begun to eliminate them naturally from your body. For a laboratory hair analysis ask your health professional or go to http://www.sanascan.com or http://www.directlabs.com

Urine Tests.
Aside from manipulating urine tests to hide drug use, a person can learn a great deal from the contents of their urine. Urine contains by-products of many chemical reactions occurring in the body that may indicate precursors to kidney disease or hypoglycemia. Urine tests being used to screen for cancer is a possibility raised by recent work of Yinfa Ma, a chemistry professor at Truman State University in Kirksville, Mo.
http://whyfiles.org/shorties/urine_test.html
Visit Direct labs http://www.directlabs.com and add Urine to your Wellness profile blood work request. You receive a kit and take the urine samples to the blood drawing facility or mail it to a pre-specified lab.

Fecal testing
The Comprehensive Digestive Stool Analysis (CDSA) is the original noninvasive evaluation of gastrointestinal function that includes analyses of digestion, absorption, bacterial balance, yeast and parasites. This profile is recommended for those with diffuse and nonspecific GI-related symptoms, such as indigestion, dysbiosis, constipation, and diarrhea. Seehttp://www.directlabs.com

Smokers Testing

The "*SmokerTest®*" offers you:
* detection of lung cancers before the appearance of any clinical sign or radiological procedures
* faster diagnosis in the presence of an isolated symptom
* follow-up of the illness during treatment
* post-treatment relapse watch, before any clinical signs. See http://www.directlabs.com

Testing you can afford!!

Direct Labs - **Discount blood testing and evaluation.** http://www.directlabs.com

Millions of us take many supplements, but do we know which ones and how much we should take?

Direct Labs provide laboratory screening tests for individuals who desire to take charge of their own health and to assist in the prevention or early detection of disease. Direct Lab's goal is to provide low cost, high quality screening services directly and confidentially to the consumer. http://www.directlabs.com

In addition to low cost blood testing, you can learn about the **DLS/CellMate Wellness Test**, an interpretive report which does an analysis of blood test results to give you a health status through your unique biochemistry plus recommended supplements, diet and recipes.
http://www.directlabs.com

Comprehensive Wellness Profile $89 includes: lipids, cbc's thyroid + tsh, kidney, liver, glucose and more.

For faster service - mention **www.Breathing.com** and pay only $10.00 extra.

Blood test is ANSWERS ONLY. NO explanation. Get urine also for extra $$. They also have an optional full explanation of the report plus recommended diet and supplements. It is called a **Cell Mate**. I use it myself. **Direct Labs 800-908-0000** (New Orleans time zone)
 http://www.directlabs.com

Chapter 12
DETOXIFICATION

✣ Do you need to remove toxins causing a health problem?
✣ Do you feel congested from too much food, or the wrong kinds of food?
✣ Do you feel lethargic, like you need a good spring cleaning?
✣ Do you want to eliminate drug residues?
✣ Do you want to offset stress to the body after illness or hospital stay?
✣ Do you want to streamline your body processes for more energy?
✣ Do you want to assist weight loss?
✣ Do you want to clear up your skin?

The following information is suggested for general maintenance. Chemically sensitive people may need a lot more detoxification methods... or if this still finds you stuffy, sneezing, headachy and coughing, you may be chemically sensitive as well and need to see a specialist.

Toxins Run Rampant!!
According to Dr. Ted Cole of the Cole Center in Cincinnati, OH, a popular song from the 1930's told us "Life is just a bowl of cherries." In 2004, an updated version of that song might go *"Life is just a bowl of toxins."* **How is that toxicity affecting your health and your life?**

Toxic exposure is not limited to people who work in nuclear power plants or live near toxic waste dumps. Every person is constantly exposed to toxins. The average person has between 90 and 300 different toxins in their tissue. Toxin exposure actually starts

BEFORE conception. How many mothers worry about the germs on a pacifier, but think nothing of wrapping their infant in a blanket treated with harsh chemicals like brominated flame retardants and perflouorinated chemicals like ScotchGuard? What effects do chemicals such as these have on infants? What effects do chemicals such as these have on any of us? We may never know. A more precise picture of human contamination with industrial chemicals is not possible, because there are very limited requirements for conducting basic health and safety testing.

A study done by the Mount Sinai School of Medicine (available at http://www.ewg.org) identified 167 toxic chemicals in the human body. How do you define toxic? Of those 167 toxic chemicals:

76 have been identified as cancer causing agents
79 have been identified as causing birth defects and delayed development
86 have been identified as causing hormone problems
94 have been identified as causing diseases of the brain and central nervous system
77 have been identified as causing diseases of the reproductive system
82 have been identified as causing diseases of the blood and the cardiovascular system
77 have been identified as causing diseases of the immune system

According to the study, an AVERAGE person has 91 of these toxins in their tissues. Depending on where you live, or work, or go to school, you could have a lot more. And that's just the external toxins that we are exposed to every day, similar to air pollution and water pollution. But there are internal toxins as well. There are toxins in our bodies that are a natural product of life. **Free radicals are toxins that our bodies produce as a normal part of metabolism. An excess of these free radicals damage the body and cause nutritional deficiencies. <u>We create toxins when we upset the acid/base balance in our body.</u>** Most diseases are acid diseases, meaning the body fluids have turned acidic.

The most common causes of acidity are: a diet high in meats, white flour, sugar, and hydrogenated oils along with tap water.

The fewer toxins you have in your body, the healthier you will be. There are two issues to address. You need to reduce the number of toxins you are exposed to, and remove the toxins already inside of you. Mobilization and excretion are required for detoxification, and the human body has many organs that work to rid you of toxins.

The lungs offer three major methods of detoxification: impaction, sedimentation and diffusion.

Any toxin that is not expelled by these methods will enter and stay in body tissue.

The liver is the primary organ in your detox defense. The liver is involved in sugar, protein and fat metabolism, as well as storage of vitamins, removal of toxins and hormones. The skin contains Cytochrome P-450 enzymes to improve the excretion of toxins via sweat. The intestinal tract excretes toxins via stool. A normal bowel function should be 1-3 soft stools a day. **Constipation is a major problem because it allows toxins to be further reabsorbed.** Your kidneys remove water-soluble substances via the urine and it can be very sensitive to chemical damage. The lymph system acts as a "second circulatory system". It is a drainage system for the connective tissue that carries waste products and toxins to the appropriate area for excretion.

Here are other methods you can use to minimize the amount of toxins your body needs to deal with:

Therapies - Different toxins respond to different therapies. The body is faced with two choices when exposed to a toxin: eliminate it, or keep it. If it cannot be excreted, the toxin is bound to various tissues, and does not show up very well on many tests.

Some of the therapies to look for include:
- Chelation binds with metal to remove it from tissue
- Tissue Mineral Analysis gives metabolic and nutritional information
- Ozone Steam Detox is effective in removing chemicals
- Neural therapy is a method to track down noxious agents that are affecting health.
- Herbs have multiple effects and include detox, nutritional, tonic, regenerative, etc.
- Fasting can be very stressful and can make things worse, and it must be done carefully and with the right personal support.
- Hyperbaric Oxygen Therapy has significant detox effects, but cost is an issue for some
- Energetic/Emotional work
- Color therapy
- WATSU –Water shiatsu
- Acupressure
- Essential Oils are similar to herbs but are more concentrated and potent. These have effects on several areas such as detoxification, immune support, anti- infectious processes, and hormonal balance.
   See our Respiratory Enhancer
- Massage helps with lymph drainage, improves circulation and muscle tone, and decreases inflammation.

Detox should be viewed as an ongoing daily process as much as bathing and brushing one's teeth. Due to our environment, we are constantly exposed to toxins, and it is best to view this as an ongoing process. Teach your children what their home and local detoxification needs are.

Foods for Detoxification

Organic foods have less toxic loads than commercially grown foods. Frozen foods are better than foods stored in aluminum cans. **Juicing organic fruits and vegetables is nutritious and healthy**. *Avoid artificial sweeteners. Artificial sweeteners are full of chemicals that the body cannot process, and many artificial sweeteners stimulate appetite.*

Stevia , Erythritol, xylitol and aguave are good alternatives to sugar.

These foods are great for detox and safe to consume every day. Blend them altogether to taste using a new VitaMix on eBay $400.00 (or used approx $125.00). Juicing organic fruits and veggies is good also but the fiber is a better "mover" of large solid debris.

1. Apples and grapes are high in fiber to cleanse the colon. "The pectin present in apples helps detoxify the gut, while the phytonutrients in grapes support the immune system, which in turn addresses toxins in the body," says integrated-medicine specialist Elson Haas, M.D. Both fruits are easily tainted by pesticides, so buy organic when possible. (**Miracle 2 Neutralizer** is a good wash for produce because it neutralizes pesticides and herbicides.)

2. Artichokes are a source of antioxidants and liver-supporting cynarin. "Artichoke not only cleanses the liver," says holistic nutritionist Ann Louise Gittleman, Ph.D., "but also helps convert the inactive T 4 thyroid hormone to an active T3, which helps to increase metabolism and weight loss. Artichoke also helps the liver decongest fats."

3. Cranberries kill bacteria in the urinary tract and contain diges-tive enzymes that cleanse the lymphatic system, says Gittleman. Unsweetened cranberry juice is available at health-food stores.

4. Leafy greens like chard, kale, spinach, dandelions, chickweed, and salad leaves not only are among the most nutrient-rich vegetables, they help purify the GI tract. Buy organic-or collect fresh greens from untreated soil.

5. Lemons contain antioxidant, antiseptic, and cleansing substances. Once ingested, lemon's alkaline effect helps counter excess acid, while its high vitamin-C content bolsters the immune system.

6. Whey, a milk protein that's rich in amino acids, offers immune-system and bone support. Research has shown it also helps the body pro-duce more glutathione, facilitating toxin removal. Suggest you get undenatured whey power which needs refrigeration.

HERBS FOR DETOXIFICATION

Your detox plan should support the organs and systems that naturally neutralize and eliminate toxins. These botanicals offer a good start:

Schisandra (Schisandra chinensis), a Chinese tonic herb, is a multitasker. "It's an antioxidant, an anti-inflammatory, a liver protector-they keep finding out more about it," notes Tilgner. Chew the berries, drink the tea, or take 10 to 50 drops of tincture, up to four times a day. (Talk to your doctor if you have high blood pressure.)

Burdock (Ardium lappa), the cleansing herb of our grandparents, can today back up its traditional use with research. It helps protect the liver and clears toxins that lead to skin eruptions like eczema and acne. Cook with the root, or take 20 to 40 drops of tincture up to four times a day.

Milk thistle (Silybum marianum), known for centuries as a liver cleanser, has been clinically shown to increase levels of glutathione, the amino-acid compound that's necessary for toxin removal. Take a teaspoon or two of the ground seeds twice a day, or ingest it as a tea or tincture, or in capsules, according to package instructions.

Sylimarin, which is a complex of flavolignans, is another option.)

Licorice (Cilycyrrhiza glabra) supports the liver, the adrenals, and the immune system. It also acts as a gentle laxative. Take it as a tea or tincture according to package instructions. Licorice may not be appropriate for patients with high blood pressure, so consult your doctor before using it if you are at risk.

Dandelion (Taraxacum officinalis) stimulates the gallbladder, the kidneys (as a diuretic), arid the liver, increasing bile production. The more bitter, the better, advises herbalist Sharol Tilgner, N.D., at least in terms of increasing the liver's ability to function optimally. Harvest some fresh, or purchase as a tea.

ENVIRONMENT

The average person breathes 150 pounds of particles and toxins per year. HEPA filters are OK, but a negative ION filter and/or an electrostatic filter in the house provides the best quality air. Negative ION generators bind with particles in the air and remove them. Avoid being around tobacco smoke.

HOME, OFFICE, OUTSIDE

Home can be a major source of toxic exposure. There are simple things you can do to eliminate some of the toxins. Reduce exposure to toxic chemicals by eliminating synthetic air fresheners, cleaning agents that contain ammonia, or chlorine, dryer softener sheets, pest control sprays, and chemical based lawn services from your home .

Geopathic stress can be toxic to the body. To reduce toxic exposure, use a headset rather than pressing your cell phone to your head. Choose a watch that winds or self winder rather than a watch with a battery. Be aware of things that may interfere with your electromagnetic field (microwaves, wireless phones, power lines, electric blankets, some computers, etc). Don't forget about your emotional/energetic environment. Your relationships with friends, the boss, your job, fellow employees, and social groups can be toxic. This will eventually affect the physical body. . Get Debra Dadd's book: The Non Toxic Home

Taking a hot shower in regular chlorinated tap water exposes you to vaporized chlorine, which is highly toxic. An inexpensive shower filter from http://www.ionlight.com will make your morning shower healthier. Skin brushing replenishes and invigorates the skin. Antibacterial soap does not make you cleaner or healthier. Glycerin soaps are a great toxin-free alternative. Avoid deodorants containing aluminum and propylene glycol and toothpastes containing sodium laurel sulfate (it foams) and fluoride. Use makeup that is non-toxic. Avoid parabens and ethylene glycol, and avoid toxic hair color, perms, etc.

TOXIC HOUSEHOLD CLEANERS

The average house-hold stores 3 to 25 gallons of toxic materials, mostly in the form of cleaning supplies. Some have been linked to cancer, asthma, liver or brain damage. Remove products with labels reading "warning," "danger," or "poison" to a hazardous waste facility.

Eliminate anything containing alcohol, ammonia, chlorine, formaldehyde, acids, lye, or propellants. This includes powder cleanser and all -purpose spray cleaner, both of which usually contain bleach, and ammonia-based glass cleaner. (Even in small amounts, bleach and ammonia can irritate your eyes, skin, nose, and throat.) Substitute plant-based products such as those made by Ecover and Mrs. Meyer's.

Natural disinfectants and cleaners like borax and vinegar also work well.

(from Jan Jenson @ *The WELLth Coach!*:)
- **Miracle 2 products** are fabulous and have all sorts of practical and life-saving uses! They are liquid cleansers made without chemicals of any kind. They work better than the toxic stuff normally found in stores and the ingredients are entirely from plant sources.
- Each of these products are so free of toxic substances of any kind, you can drink them without ill effect!
- As a matter of fact, taken internally in small amounts, these Miracle II Soaps are very effective at detoxing the body.

- Sounds too good to be true ... <u>an industrial-strength, multi-purpose cleanser that will meet all your personal care and household needs.</u> These inspired, concentrated formulas are made from all-natural ingredients and will clean, degrease and deodorize anything, from your glass and mirrors, carpet and upholstery and even heavy cleaning such as grease traps and oil spots on the concrete garage floor, to your baby's bottom.
- **These Miracle 2 Soaps form a toxin-cleansing system**. No fragrances in them. Totally safe around small children and pets. In fact, my cat won't drink water without Neutralizer!
- **The basis of Miracle 2's function is pH balance**, alkalinity; not only in the human body, but
also applicable in agriculture, bringing our soured soils back to alkaline balance. Major reports
from worldwide growers are attracting more agricultural application, which can help millions.

If you would like to order Miracle 2 products: http://www.global-light-network.com/store/shopaff.asp? affid=364

TOLL FREE order line: **1-888-236-2108**   Use Affiliate ID #364

PESTICIDES

Studies have linked pesticides to cancer, birth defects, infertility, and damage to the cen-tral nervous system. Kill cock-roaches, ants, and termites by dusting borax in suspect areas. For major ant infestations, mix borax and water with a little sugar (for sugar ants) or grease (for grease ants). Safety note: Though it's natu-ral and relatively safe, borax is not entirely non toxic so keep it away from food, children and pets. Vacuuming regularly also holds down the dust mite and creepy crawler population.

CHEMICAL LEFTOVERS

Another name for old paint and stains, motor oil, batteries, thinners, and solvents is toxic trash. These have chemicals that, when disposed of unsafely, can injure sanitation workers, contaminate septic tanks or wastewater treatment systems, and pollute ground and surface water.

Deliver them to a hazardous- waste drop-off center. Call your city's sanitation department for the location of your nearest site. The EPA also offers information about disposal and recycling on its Web site (epa.gov). If you have enough paints or stains left over, see if you can give them to a neighbor, charity, or business who will use them.

DEAD TECHNOLOGICAL EQUIPMENT

One computer can contain 5 to 8 pounds of lead. Turn to the people who made it or sold it. **Office Depot** (http://www.officedepot.com) allows customers to bring one item per visit for recycling — a monitor, printer, or cell-phone, for example. Most large computer companies like **Dell** (http://www.dell.com), **Epson** (funding factory. com), and **Hewlett-Packard** (http://www.hp.com) offer recycling programs.

PAPER PILES

Recycle what you're never to read. Preventive maintenance: remove your name from junk mail lists by con-tacting the Mail Preference Service http://www.dmaconsumers.org/consumerassistance.html Cancel catalogs and magazines you never look at. Sign up to pay bills online.

Toss old flour and rice products that can develop bugs. If there's no expiration date and you can't remember when you bought it get rid of it. Keep new products fresh and bug-free in the freezer!

FLOORS. Carpeting is a magnet for mold, mites, dust, and the toxins tracked in from the outside. I prefer wood floors and throw rugs. If you don't have a HEPA filter on your vacuum cleaner, as much as 70 per-cent of the dirt might be coming right back out of the bag. Vacuum car-pets weekly (daily in high traffic spots like entryways) in each direc-tion.

Cleaning bare non wood floors

1.25 cup vinegar per 1 quart water
On wood; plain hot water on marble, tile, and granite (cleaners will pit them); and hot water and a little dish soap. Weekly if no heavy traffic.

BATHROOM
Fungi, a major source of allergens. Wipe down the walls and curtain once a week. Mix borax, vinegar, and hot water. Use Miracle 2 moisturizing soap in the shower. It leaves little or no scum.

FIREPLACE
Remove spent ashes. Add them to your com-post heap. Ashes are too alkaline for the garden. Clean chimney once a year. Fireplaces can generate carbon monoxide, and creosote buildup can create a fire hazard.

WINDOWS
Mix 3 tablespoons vinegar, 1/2 teaspoon liquid soap, and 2 cups warm water in a spray bottle. Spray and wipe with a squeegee, going over the edges with cotton rags.

MAJOR SPOTS — MAKE SURE THEY ARE CLEAN!
- Sink and cutting boards
- Your kitchen sink can have more bacteria than your toilet bowl. Yech!
- Pantry
- Twice yearly take every single thing out and vacuum the crumbs. Then wash the shelves with borax-
- Refrigerator
- Dump mysterious stuff molding at the back of the fridge. Wipe the shelves with a disinfecting blend of 1 teaspoon borax, 3 tablespoons vinegar, and 2 cups hot water from a spray bottle. Try using 3% food grade hydrogen peroxide for mold that causes smells and spoils food faster.

SWEATING AND DETOXIFICATION.
Saunas and steam baths have been used for centuries by cultures around the world to bring about detoxification and better health. Traditionally, saunas have been used to improve mental clarity, to

diminish pain, and to promote longevity. From Finland to Native America, the sauna/sweat room and sweat lodges have been a tradition for centuries or more.

There are TWO kinds of "sweat rooms". One is in a wooden or tented sweat lodge room with hot rocks and steam and the other is a wooden room using the equivalent of the suns heating (not the burning ones as in ultraviolet but the warming infrared ones) rays. I've been in and love both but the Far Infrared version warms deeper and faster, is more convenient, cheaper to operate, portable and may be installed in any room in the house by assembling it in an hour and plugging it in.

Your lungs are a critical aspect of natural detoxification. Internal cleansing is mandatory for optimal respiratory maintenance. The sauna causes massive sweating. On top of the daily oxy-cleanse ingestion you must sweat as much as you can. Just make sure you replace the water and the sodium via sea salt.

Far-Infrared (FIR) heat is a form of naturally occurring energy that directly heats objects by gentle infrared radiation heat, rather than by raising the temperature of the surrounding air. FIR heat is completely safe for the human body. Physical therapists often use FIR heat to promote healing, and hospitals use the same heat to keep premature babies warm in incubators.

In the past few years, hyperthermic (sweat) therapy has been studied extensively. Through this research, it has been shown that far infrared saunas greatly assist in the elimination of accumulated toxins due to the deep level therapeutic heating. Toxic metals and waste such as mercury, lead, nickel, cadmium, alcohol, nicotine, sodium and cholesterol are excreted in high quantities in the sweat during a 30-min infrared sauna session.

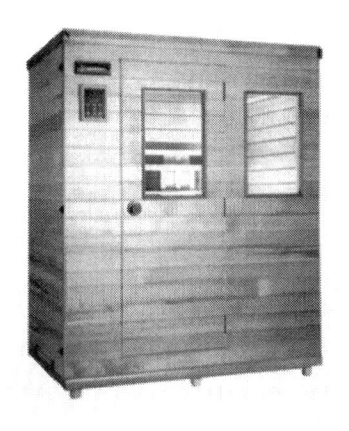

Sweating also reduces stress and fatigue; burns calories, reduces cellulite, helps control weight; removes toxins and wastes;

relaxes and soothes muscles. It relieves pain and joint stiffness; boosts metabolism and improves the immune system. It also promotes a healthier skin condition and skin tone; enhanced blood circulation, and gives you a gentle but effective cardiovascular workout.

Do not be fooled by non-ceramic heaters. The best FIR saunas use ceramic heaters, with 16 minerals in the ceramic which produce therapeutic far infrared waves. The non-ceramic heaters produce only heat, not infrared waves. There are many phony FIR saunas on the market. I saw one (a $600.00 canvas version) being sold at a Conference in Los Angeles.

SAUNA EXERCISE:

During a 10-20 minute FIR sauna session, your heart rate increases by 50-75%. This provides the same metabolic result as physical exercise. The increased cardiac load is the equivalent to a brisk walk. There is a nominal effect on blood pressure because the heat also causes blood vessels in skin to expand to accommodate increased blood flow. To repeat. Those that do not or can not exercise can still receive incredible self healing benefits for regular FIR sauna sweats.

DETOXIFICATION:

Toxins such as sodium, alcohol, nicotine, cholesterol and carcinogenic heavy metals (cadmium, lead, zinc, nickel) accumulate in the body during modern daily life. The body eliminates most toxins naturally by sweating. Heat therapy stimulates the sweat glands that cleanse and detoxify the skin. The heat simply speeds up the body's natural process. Those that do not or can not exercise can still receive incredible self healing benefits.

PAIN RELIEF:

Heat relieves pain by expanding blood vessels and increasing circulation. Better circulation allows more oxygen to reach injured areas of the body and helps reduce pain and speed up the healing process.

WEIGHT CONTROL:
Perspiring is part of the complex thermoregulatory process of the body that increases the heart rate, cardiac output, and metabolic rate. The process requires a large amount of energy and reduces excess moisture, salt and subcutaneous fat. Fat becomes water-soluble and the body sweats out fats and toxins.

INDUCED FEVER:
During a fever, the body heats up to eliminate viruses and attack foreign agents. This rise in temperature is a natural stage of the immune system's healing process and is one of the best ways to rid the body of chemicals and unwelcome visitors. The combination of heat, extra water and the immune system weakens the hold of viruses and bacterial growth. Saunas induce an "artificial fever" by heating up the body but without the pains of an illness. Subsequently, the body wards off invading organisms much more easily because the immune system is activated consistently by the "artificial fever". More about FIR saunas at http://www.breathing.com/sauna.htm

For more about detoxification go to http://www.TheWellthRevolution.com and let Jan Jenson keep you up to date.

Below are some good web site related to detoxification and toxic drug side effects:
http://www.ciin.org/
http://www.pesticide.org
http://www.iceh.org
http://www.rachel.org
http://www.sehn.org
http://www.sustainer.org
http://www.garynull.com/documents/prozac1.htm
http://www.garynull.com/documents/prozac2.htm
http://www.quitpaxil.org
http://www2.netdoor.com/~bill/prosurv/prosurv.html
http://www.alternativementalhealth.com/default_1.htm
http://www.breggin.com/
http://www.prozacbacklash.com/

CHAPTER 13
Cleansing, Fasting

INTERNAL CLEANSING

Clean healthy bodies use oxygen more effectively when they are not full of waste. Cleansing removes debris and increases oxygen utilization, as the waste would sidestep oxygen in its normal cell building duties. Continued slowness of elimination can cause toxic buildup and strain the organs of elimination. Fiber serves to push or carry waste and undigested food through the intestines. Without it, putrefaction of stagnating nutrients and waste products occurs causing a diverting of the available health producing oxygen supply to neutralize excess bacteria and pathogens.

A "backed up" large or small intestine often causes bad breath. Clean your colon and your gums may stop bleeding.

The Common Cold

Colds are the body's attempt to rid itself of toxins and debris, a cleansing reaction. They are largely due to a backup of the large intestine, too much mucous producing foods, too little water in the diet, and often precipitated by stress in the form of a rapid change of season most often experienced in the Summer-Autumn transition.

Climactic changes are a form of stress; they induce an increase in the hormone cortisol, which in turn depresses immunity and increases susceptibility to infections. The stress modulating power of balanced breathing can reduce cortisol production and help maintain the body's "inner heat".

My son used to have a cold for two weeks when he lived in New York. He came to live with me in San Francisco and the cold lasted but ONE day. First sign of sniffles I kept him in bed, omitted food, gave him a cathartic such as Exlax, had him drink 2 quarts of fresh grapefruit juice fortified with 15 grams per quart of powdered vitamin C, enough to last him 24 hours or more. When he wasn't in bed he was on the toilet. ONE DAY.

Detoxification is the normal body process of eliminating or neutralizing toxins through the colon, liver, kidneys, lungs, lymph and skin. Fasting is the world's most ancient and natural healing mechanism. Fasting triggers a truly wondrous cleansing process that reaches right down to each and every cell and tissue in the body. **Therapeutic fasting and detoxification are two major methods of internal cleansing which help produce optimal health through natural hygiene. Studies show that many other animal species are smart enough to do their own fasting for health benefits.**

Here's what a few "experts" in the field of fasting have to say about the effects of proper, regular fasting and cleansing:

Evart Loomis M.D. -*"Fasting is the world's most ancient and natural healing mechanism. Fasting triggers a truly wondrous cleansing process that reaches right down to each and every cell and tissue in the body. Within 24 hours of curtailing food intake, enzymes stop entering the stomach and travel instead into the intestines and into the bloodstream, where they circulate and gobble up all sorts of waste matter, including dead and damaged cells, unwelcome microbes, metabolic wastes, and pollutants. All organs and glands get a much needed and well-deserved rest, during which their tissues are purified and rejuvenated and their functions balanced and regulated. The entire alimentary canal is swept clean. By rebuilding immunity, health is naturally restored and disease disappears. If health and immunity are thereafter conscientiously maintained, the individual is no longer vulnerable to disease and dieting become unnecessary. Surely one of the most overlooked and yet most valuable modes of healing that will be rediscovered in the future of the new medicine is the fast. This is because of the increasing* interest in looking to oneself for healing powers. For the fast is an inward process and cannot be entered upon only from an outer approach with any expectation of a lasting benefit. The person must invariably be involved with the overall results. This therapeutic encounter is in direct contrast to the usual non-involvement in the physician-directed, disease-oriented medical practice of today."

Patricia Bragg Ph.D.- Daughter of Paul Bragg. *"Proven throughout history for physical, mental and spiritual rejuvenation, fasting promotes cleansing and healing; helps normalize weight, blood pressure, cholesterol; rebuilds the immune system; and helps reverse the aging process. If we are to get these poisons out of our bodies we must fast. By fasting we give our bodies a physiological rest. This rest builds Vital Force. The more Vital Force we have, the more toxins are going to be eliminated from the body to help keep it clean, pure and healthy."*

Benjamin Franklin - *"The best of all medicines are rest and fasting."*

Dr. Herbert Shelton - *"It is estimated that fasting for the alleviation of human suffering has been practiced uninterruptedly for 10,000 years. No doubt it has been employed from the time man first began to get sick. Fasting was part of the methods of healing practiced in the Ancient Asculapian Temples of Toscurd Guido, 1300 years before the time of Jesus. Hippocrates, the mythical Greek "Father of Physic," seems to have prescribed total abstinence from food while a "disease" was on the increase, and especially at the critical period, and a spare diet on other occasions. Tertullian has left us a treatise on fasting written about 200 A.D. Plutarch said: "Instead of using medicine rather fast a day." Avicenna, the great Arab physician often prescribed fasting for three weeks or more."*

Dr. Joseph Mercola - *"We can solve well over 90% of the all chronic diseases with simple, inexpensive natural therapies. I was once a victim of the never-ending flow of propaganda from the medical establishment (which I think of as the "disease" establishment because they focus on disease rather than on prevention and wellness) who wants to maintain a monopoly on the word "cure" and who wants us to believe that we have no* *control over our own health and that our only hope to get "well" is with drugs, surgery and radiation "First do no harm..."*

Elimination of the symptom is NOT the same as elimination of the disease.

The fastest way to restore wellness is to stop putting into the body the things that have caused the physical problem to develop in the first place, and then give the body the nutrients it needs to repair and rebuild itself. The holistic approach treats the whole person, ignites the body's internal healing force and stimulates the body's natural abilities to heal itself.

There are, of course, some potential dangers while fasting, though they are few and far between. There are many symptoms which may arise while fasting, and a few that almost certainly will: lowered blood pressure, lowered body temperature, and coated tongue.

Blood pressure is virtually guaranteed to drop while fasting, and will stay lower if intelligent lifestyle choices are followed after the fast. This is great news for the 50% of Americans who will die of the ravages of high-blood pressure, heart disease, or stroke. It's worth noting for all fasters because below-normal blood pressure, while not inherently dangerous or problematic often results in orthostatic hypotension (standing up too fast and getting dizzy, in English).

Rest assured, that fasting - done properly - provides the body with the optimal conditions which to heal itself, and there is nothing better you could do for yourself.

FASTING

4 major styles.
1. Nothing at all.
2. Water.
3. Juices.
4. Vegetable broths and juices.
Each has it benefits and advocates.

1. Fasting using no water, fruits juices or anything.
This is pretty radical to me and I have only met one person that advocated it. He was a PhD from Russia and a very sturdy fellow. I can't say he is wrong but I have not heard very much about that so I am naturally cautious and advise against it unless you have some very careful blood work pre-testing and fasting supervision.

2. Water Fasting
The water fast is well represented. Loren Lockman at the Tanglewood wellness center in Maryland
and Costa Rica. Loren is one of the very best and a trusted colleague. Below follows a recap of a
water fast.

Near-Death to Amazing Health in One Week

At the time I met Jim, he was suffering from congestive heart failure, type two diabetes, gout, hypertension, high cholesterol, inability to sleep more than two hours, (and only in one position), and numerous conditions related to diabetes, including progressive loss of eyesight and scaly skin all over his face, torso, arms and legs. He was unable to walk more than about 100 yards because he was in so much pain, and was taking 17 different medications every day. He weighed 340 pounds, (which would have been the ideal weight for him – if he were about 14 feet tall!) Jim's doctor had exhausted conventional treatment options, and told him that he had only weeks to live, and that maybe I could help him.

During our first consultation, (which lasted 3 hours), I told Jim what he needed to do in order to stay alive for the next couple of weeks, and that he needed to clear his schedule for at least a month to fast. He informed me that at the CEO of two corporations, he couldn't afford to take that much time off. I reminded him that, according to his doctor, he was likely to be dead within a month or two. He finally agreed to fast for one week. Priorities.

I had a conference call with his internist and his cardiologist and explained that I needed Jim off all of his medications prior to fasting. His internist said: "We can't take him off his diabetes medication." "Oh," I said, "why not?" "Because he'll go into diabetic shock, coma. He could die." "Well," I said, I'm not the doctor, but my experience is that when we simply get out of the way, it takes care of itself."

Next his cardiologist spoke up. "We can't take him off his hypertension medications." "Oh, " I said, "how come?" "Because his blood pressure will skyrocket. It could kill him," the doctor replied. "Well, " I said again, " You guys are the experts, but I've found that if we just get out of the way, it seems to take care of itself."

They agreed to take Jim off all medications, and though I like to think that I'm pretty persuasive, I don't kid myself that I convinced these two doctors of anything. Rather, I suspect that they figured Jim was going to die pretty soon, and they might as well allow him to die at my place rather than under their care.

So Jim came to the center and commenced his fast. Within 24 hours of initiating his fast, Jim was able to read the newspaper for the first time in months.

After 48 hours of fasting, the gout in his legs was gone, both legs completely cleared of fluid. Jim had spent much of the first two days standing in front of the toilet urinating away the excess water that mega-doses of diuretics couldn't eliminate. The difference was simple: having eliminated the stored uric acid, his body no longer needed the water to buffer his system, and the excess water was simply and naturally peed away. Over the next couple of days, we watched Jim continue to improve, eliminating one symptom after another. On the fifth day, we took a blood sugar reading, and his blood sugar was normal. This is remarkable only because he had not been able to achieve a normal blood sugar reading with 6 years of medication.

By the time Jim completed his 7 day fast, he was sleeping through the night for the first time in years, his skin had cleared completely, and he was feeling better than he had in years. This man, who hadn't been able to walk more than 100 yards prior to his fast, walked half a mile after seven days of fasting, before his first meal!

In fact, virtually every one of Jim's conditions had completely resolved within seven days; his hypertension was the only exception. As typically happens with people with a significant degree of plaque in their arteries, Jim's blood pressure had risen slightly early in the fast, and had descended below his starting point. One week simply wasn't long enough to resolve this most-important issue. Still, by giving is body the opportunity to really cleanse and heal itself, Jim went from seventeen medications to one.

Jim's story is amazing not because of the results he achieved, but rather because those results were achieved in only 7 days. At Tanglewood, we see these kind of "miracles" all the time, they just usually take a bit longer to manifest. http://www.tanglewoodwellnesscenter.com/testimonials/stories_jim.php
Paul Bragg was a staunch advocate of water fasting and wrote an excellent book about it called ***The Miracle of Fasting.***

Arnold Ehret wrote a great book called ***Rational Fasting***. A must read.

3. Juices
The Master Cleanser is a good fast using primarily lemon juice.
Norman Walker, who invented the Norwalk Juicer wrote several books about juice fasting or juicing for health and longevity. He lived to age 118.
Fresh Vegetable and Fruit Juices is one of my favorites — any book by Walker is a good buy.

4. Veggie Broths.
Paavo Airolia called his fasting juice fasting but they were mostly combinations of boiled veggies into a fiberless broth taken with water and some juices.
I began my first fast using Paavo's How to Keep Slim, Healthy and Young With Juice Fasting. It was fantastic.
Use our nasal washing device to help clear the sinuses from bacteria and dried mucous.. www.breathing.com/sinu-cleanse.htm.

HERBAL DETOXIFICATION
By Ted H. Spence, DDS, ND, PhD/DSc, MPH

Generic diets for detoxification are good, but may not stimulate the liver, lungs or the kidneys as much as one would like.

Therefore, herbal cleanses are indicated when we want to hone our cleanse to a "*sharp edge*" and be organ specific. Of course, herbs are foods too and provide one with vitamins, minerals and enzymes for excellent nutrition. Herbs are powerful, because they may be combined together to fortify those herbs that aid specific organs. For example, herbal combinations that aid the liver may be found in many organic food stores. The following list shows how herbal combinations help the various organs.

Herbal Combinations
Liver
LIV-A Dandelion, red beet, liverwort, parsley, horsetail, birch leaves, chamomile, blessed thistle, black cohosh, angelica, gentian, goldenrod

Kidneys
Uva ursi, parsley, dandelion, juniper berries JP-X, parsley, uva ursi, marshmallow, ginger, goldenseal, dong
quai, cedar berries

Lungs
LH Comfrey, marshmallow, mullein, slippery elm, senega,, Chinese ephedra

While herbs may be taken at any time, they are best for detoxification purposes when they are used with a good diet. It does not make any sense to take herbs to cleanse the liver if the bowels are clogged with junk or refined foods, since the liver dumps its toxins into the bowels. And while detoxification diets are effective by themselves, they may be reinforced and speeded up with herbs, which stimulate the eliminative organs.

 Herbs may be used as teas, powders or extracts. Powders are usually encapsulated for easier swallowing, but are best when taken with meals and digestive enzymes. Extracts may be used when specific herbs are needed, but may be extracted with alcohol, which we need to avoid. Herbal teas are easily made and easily taken all throughout the day. They are mild and gentle and sometimes refreshing and sometimes bitter. Experimentation may be in order until one develops the right tea to drink. Herbal teas is a topic in itself, since there are so many and different ways to make them.

Pathogens

Viruses, including cancer, molds and bacteria, will reduce oxygen utilization and make the lungs work harder to compensate for other malfunctioning body systems. They cannot survive as well or at all in a high oxygen environment. Ask your health professional for an appropriate blood test or get one direct from http://www.directlabs.com

Parasites

Parasites overtake the energy-making centers of our cells using the oxygen we need to maintain good health and to reproduce them. Allergies obstruct our airways and deprive cells of oxygen.. Parasites produce free radicals that attack cell membranes and the mitochondrial furnaces of the cells, making it more difficult for oxygen to get into the cells where it can fuel the energy process. Better add to your parasite program http://www.huldaclark.com and her inexpensive program of cloves, wormwood and walnut hull tincture plus her zapper.

Parasite removal programs include die-off as well and can cost as much as $800. See our Parasite Assessment Questionnaire in our 32 page Holistic Health Assessment included FREE in our #250 and weight loss program: http://www.breathing.com/weight-loss-program.htm

Environmental and psychological stressors debilitate both the "outer" breathing of the lungs and the "inner" breathing of the cells.

Ask your health professional for a stool test from **Great Smokey's Laboratory** http://www.gsmcweb.com or get one from http://www.directlabs.com and/or one of the many tests at http://www.directlabs.com/testtypes.php#DMSP

During a fast the nervous system gets a chance to rest. Because breathing drives the nervous system like a wagon master drive a team of horses, if the breathing is out of balance it will greatly impede the efficiency of rest. I strongly encourage breathing development during a fast. It will accelerate all benefits when done accurately and systematically.

CANDIDA is a parasite

Better breathing will help rid you of candida but do not expect it to have to work alone or even do the major portion of the work.

If you suspect you may have candida see our Candida assessment Questionnaire in our 32 page **Holistic Health Assessment** included FREE in many of our programs including the Weight Loss program. http://www.breathing.com/weight-loss-program.htm

"Cofactors in oxygen utilization decrease Candida yeast and all Yeast strengthening substances." Dr. Crook The Yeast Connection

Candida will steal your breath, your energy, and your life. Yeast is found in minute quantities along with millions of beneficial B vitamin producing bacteria (Lactobacilli) in a healthy body.

Candida is a dimorphic organism, having the chameleon-like ability to change from yeast to the mycelial fungal form. The yeast-like form is a noninvasive, sugar-fermenting organism. The fungal form produces rhitzoids, long root-like structures that are invasive and can penetrate the intestinal mucosa like in "leaky gut" syndrome, releasing metabolic toxins, and incompletely digested proteins into the blood stream. This initiates a series of adverse reactions that may cause tissue damage, and a wide range of problems, including food sensitivities and allergies.

HOW DOES CANDIDA MULTIPLY AND TAKE OVER?

❏Antibiotics kill off the beneficial bacteria, which normally suppress Candida. Mutant or wild type bacteria are created which are highly resistant to antibiotics.

❏ Nutritional Deficiencies, Poor diet, poor digestion and mal-absorption from gluten intolerance all set the stage for poor resistance to Candida overgrowth.

❏ Antibiotic Residues in Commercial Meat: We encourage antibiotic and hormone-free meats.
Use of Recreational Drugs, Alcohol, Marijuana, Cocaine, Heroin, Tobacco, etc., these drugs stresses the liver, adrenals, and the immune system and decreases the resistance to Candida.
❏The Pill. The hormones in birth control pills encourage yeast growth. Cortisone, Prednisone, etc. encourage yeast growth.
❏Operations, Catheterization, Radiation, Anti-Cancer Drugs, Amalgam Fillings: Some holistic practitioners feel the leaching of mercury from silver/mercury amalgams puts a toxic load on the body, preventing full health and complete eradication of Candida.
❏ Anti-yeast Pharmaceuticals, including Oral and Topical Preparations are producing new resistant strains of these microorganisms. This can lead to recurrent infections that resist treatment and become a debilitating health problem.
❏ Reduced oxygen supplies: Oxygen will help kill germs, bacteria, virus and fungus. Candida is a fungus. Having adequate oxygen stores reduces biochemical stresses and maximizes bodily function in the presence of parasites such as Candida.

WHO CAN GET CANDIDA?

Men, Women, children, elderly, pregnant women (due to hormonal changes, stress and higher nutrient needs often not met), all are candidates for getting Candida. The yeast needs food, water, warmth and darkness. The yeast typically starts growing in the intestinal tract and spills over into the reproductive area.
Note: I've read that the Spermicide Noxynol-9 kills healthy bacteria in the female reproductive system.

WHAT HAPPENS?

Candida often first spreads in the Gastrointestinal tract and many symptoms can develop, such as gas, bloating, indigestion, heartburn, nausea, constipation and/or diarrhea, and major cravings for sugar, starches and alcohol, which are the foods the Candida increasingly demands. The more Candida foods that are consumed the worse you begin to feel, as Candida proliferates, releasing toxins and interfering with digestion.
Eventually, the yeast enters the blood stream and spreads through

the body. At this point, the immune system begins to be overwhelmed and to falter. As the Candida spreads, symptoms grow more diffuse and convoluted: Depression, lethargy, mental confusion/fog, mood swings, PMS, confused thyroid function, susceptibility to infections (sinus, respiratory, bladder, gums, etc.), sensitivity to pollutants, fumes (which can become full-blown "environmental illness"), achy muscles and/or joints, skin fungus...

WHAT IS RECOMMENDED?

Extensive research shows that a successful program for controlling Candida and fungal overgrowth must achieve three goals. **First**, the Candida and fungal population of the body must be gradually, yet significantly reduced. **Second**, the immune system must be strengthened, and activated to further deplete Candida or fungal overgrowth. **Third**, the health of the intestinal tract must be rebuilt. This may be accomplished through re-seeding the colon with friendly flora, and by normalizing the pH of the gastrointestinal tract. -

Proper breathing: The way we breathe dictates oxygen quantity and nervous system balance. Unbalanced breathing will negate any attempts to maintain proper pH balance without which every biochemical reaction in the body becomes at risk.

Nutritional support, including booster foods and specific supplements for reducing Candida overgrowth, healing the intestinal tract and increasing energy such as with liquid potassium.

Eating plan: eliminating sugars, starches and alcohol strictly for two weeks, two months or forever.

Immune System Boosters: Massive immune system rebuilding; especially with chronic food/sugar/alcohol, etc. addictions.

Nutritional Yeast: An inactive yeast rich in nutrients, which also increases vitality and mental clarity.

Avoid exposure to toxins sprays, solvents, and non-organic foods. Digestive enzymes and possibly hydrochloric acid

Fiber speeds up transit time in gut to reduce putrefaction and bacteria breeding environment.

Prevent constipation even if you just know you don't have it. You probably do in a way you can't possibly tell, yet.

Exercise: The lymph doesn't move much unless you do; the legs, arms and chest expansion and contraction are the pump.

Natural Antifungals: Restoring healthy intestinal ecology with high potency Lactobacilus powders and liquids, probiotics such as garlic, ginger, oregano oil, echinacea.

Acupuncture helps restore balance to the immune system, the adrenals, digestion and elimination. Eases Detox considerably.

Keep dry'. Remember food, darkness, warmth, and moisture? Use white or rose clay powders in undergarments and between toes. Green clay powders might not wash out of clothes.

Clothing. Many synthetics trap moisture on the skin: many female undergarments, etc. Use of natural fibers, cotton and silk are recommended.

Water is used to hydrate cells and flush waste. Drink a minimum of one quart per day. Only water counts as water; not juice, coffee, etc.

The following super nutrient is highly recommended and should accelerate most regeneration programs.

Germanium in E3live or from http://www.tidhealth.com
E3live. (helps control blood sugar levels to reduce cravings for sweets.) http://www.breathing.com/e3live.htm

Breathing development, relaxation,& meditations from Breathing.com

Yoga, warm water soaking, biofeedback, massage or therapeutic touch Love - both the giving and receiving This can begin with caring for a plant or a pet. As one embarks upon the journey of recovery, independence can soften into acceptance of self and others, and also into receiving that staunch, sustaining love. Then the heart is like a warm hearth, and the immune system can rest and replenish and do its business.

Medical support: Many drugs impair digestion, proper assimilation of nutrients and growth of healthy bacteria.

WHAT IS DIE-OFF?

No fun! As the antifungal kill off and neutralize the Candida, you may need to rest more and alert family, friends and coworkers that you may be lethargic and grumpy. **There may be flu-like symptoms, headaches, and diarrhea. Cravings for sugar, starches and/or alcohol may suddenly surge.** It usually doesn't last long. If you do slip, **STAY WITH THE PROGRAM**. Even if you slip and eat something not on the diet, you haven't blown it. The supplements will still be working. Die off can begin in a day or two or in two weeks. Its course is hard to predict. The worst is usually over within 3 weeks. **Lemon water:** squeeze in half a lemon per 8 oz. water — helps you get through die off. The clinical nutritionist or natural hygienist may have additional recommendations.

IS THERE LIFE AFTER DIE-OFF?

Life, zest and mental clarity YES! With a non-bloated middle, good digestion and normal bowel function. Eventually, sweets taste too sweet. Depending on how long the Candida has been out of hand, how run down the immune system, adrenals, digestion, etc. are, it can take 16 months, but usually 23 months, to turn Candida around, and restore good health maybe for the first time in one's life!

ANTI-CANDIDA PLAN, WHAT TO AVOID

This list is indicative, not comprehensive. The books all give conflicting food recommendations. Choose the consistencies. Check with a health professional with extensive nutrition experience. .

Sweets, Candy of all kinds, sugar: white, brown, and raw. Maple syrup. Rice syrup, Sweeteners, Honey, Malt, Corn sweetener, high fructose corn syrup, Fructose, Corn syrup, Miso, Nutra-sweet, Aspartame, Saccharine Mushrooms Dairy Products: Milk, Cheese. Yeast containing foods, Alcohol containing foods.

Herb tea (except Pau D'Arco), Soy Sauce, Vinegars, Fruit*: Fruit juices, especially sweetened. Canned fruit. Oranges, bananas, grapes and dried fruit (raisins, dates, figs, etc.), Fruit juice concentrate. Starches; Grains m general, with the exception of rice, corn and millet, Bread, Cookies, Gravies, Muffins, Pancakes, Pasta, Sauces, Tapioca, Waffles, Corn chips, potato chips, French fries. Miscellaneous: Left over food in general, Lard, margarine, hydrogenated or partially vegetable oils, canola oil.

✶ In some cases fruit will not be recommended at all.

ANTI-CANDIDA EATING PLAN
What is okay to eat?

Daily for the first three months take two times three caps of **FOS** (creates unfriendly blood environment for yeast growth), **Oil of Oregano**. For the first 2 weeks the diet will consist simply of: vegetables particularly steamed or lightly saut•ed in the beginning, animal protein (ocean fish, antibiotic-free poultry, beef, lamb, pork). Fertile ranch eggs (cooked at low temperature), Spirulina, organic nuts and seeds prescribed amounts.

Legumes: 1 serving/day Quinoa, brown basmati rice, millet those not dairy intolerant can eat yogurt (encouraged) and buttermilk. Freshly prepared soups (non-cream or milk base). Flavoring: Liberal amounts of fresh lemon (helps with Detox). Fresh herbs rather than dried (due to mold content in dried). Garlic, onion, curry, pepper (in moderation) Oils: Flax, Olive, borage, grape or sesame seed or sesame. Vegetable juices, other liquids: Fresh carrot (small amounts 2 oz. or less due to high sugar content), celery and/or parsley juice. Lemon water before meals Water: preferably spring or filtered 6 to 8 glasses a day, 1/2 hour before meals, or I hour after Pau D 'Arco or spearmint tea

After the first 2 weeks: The diet expands gradually under the supervision of the nutritionist. Alcohol, sugar and some other substances are never reintroduced. Emphasis on foods known to have anti-fungal properties such as garlic, onions, broccoli, cabbage, kale, collards, Brussels sprouts, olive and flax oils, cinnamon and lots of cloves.

Problems still?

FAST with only WATER!

Do the OBR's, Strapping Techniques in DVD/Video **#176, Reflexive Breathing** to increase yeast and fungus killing oxygen and rebalance your nervous system. http://www.breathing.com/video-strap.htm

FOODS for cleansing the lungs and to return to good health

Useful foods are watercress, watermelon -eat an entire one by yourself, cantaloupe, apple, persimmon, peach, pear, strawberry, citrus, seaweed's, mushroom, Daiken, radish, carrot, flax seeds, pumpkin, kuzu, broccoli, parsley, kale, turnip, mustard greens, cabbage, bok choy, cauliflower, chard, papaya, and strawberries, white fungus.

Majority of diet should be in the form of **soups**. Soups and congees of millet, barley or rice are cooling and soothing for the lung heat. Add powdered flax seeds for colon cleansing.

At least two bowel movements per day or enemas to replace the BM(s) you missed. In the Boy Scouts we called toilet paper KYBO tickets. It stood for Keep Your Bowels Open. This is an ABSOLUTE MUST that will be replaced some day with adequate probiotics and healthy intestinal flora...

If you won't do enemas or colonics you'd better take some herbal cathartics or Epsom salts.

HERBS. Horehound leaf, chickweed, Pau D'arco or fresh ginger tea

HOMEOPATHY   http://www.breathing.com/8/kb.htm

CLEANSE: cleanse, cleanse, including colonic irrigation, watermelon binges, liver & kidney detoxification, and fresh juice fasts etc. Take the elimination load off the lungs as much as possible.

Meditators sitting on zafus in what looks to be an erect posture can restrict their breathing. Any repeated activity may in some way restrict one's breathing or assist it depending on how it is performed.

FOOD ALLERGY MEANS YOUR BODY REACTS TO CERTAIN FOODS

Food allergy means that your body reacts to certain foods. It is also called food hypersensitivity. Common symptoms are itching and burning around the mouth, asthma and vomiting. About 90 per cent of allergies are caused by nuts, eggs, milk or soy. Food allergies are on the increase in Western society.

Food allergies tend to occur in children under five years of age. They often have eczema and a family history of asthma and/or eczema. Food allergy is not a common cause of adverse reactions to food in adults.

Food intolerance is much more common than food allergy. It occurs as a result of a pharmacological reaction after eating or drinking, rather than an immune response which is the case with a food allergy. It has very similar symptoms to a food allergy and often it is difficult to distinguish between the two. Usually, the onset of symptoms from food intolerance is more delayed in comparison to a more immediate response from food allergies.

I see no practical difference between labeling someone allergic or sensitive, though allergic may have more health risk connected with it. They seem too close to the same - and neither is good. I suspect "sensitive" is a precursor to allergy, such as hypoglycemia is a precursor to diabetes. They BOTH need to be eliminated to acheive optimal breathing.

MIKE WHITE'S CLEANSING STORY AND RECOMMENDATIONS

My blood oxygen, as measured with a Pulse Oximeter, increased two percentage points within 2 days after the cleanse. http://www.breathing.com/articles/liver-cleanse.htm Weeks later it was the same increase without exercise. Gladly I can now refocus on my walking, weight training and breathing exercising as I had purposefully neglected them to better isolate the liver cleanse and liquid oxygen influences.

Next to and sometimes even senior to eliminating shortness of breath or other breathing restrictions, the liver cleanse has to be almost always second on my list of accelerated healing methods.

The following is a public domain article modified by me to better relate to breathing.

LIVER CLEANSE - Long Accepted by Many Natural Hygienists

When the liver is dysfunctional it puts stress on all systems. The liver is a primary organ of detoxification. So is the breath and so is the colon and kidneys. Toxins that the liver is supposed to but does not address end up in the lungs, kidneys, lymphatic system and colon. The colon will reabsorb them if they are not eliminated from the body within hours of their arrival. Once the lymphatic system gets saturated with toxins it takes perhaps weeks to remove them as the lymph is very dense and moves very slowly. Toxins reduce oxygen supply which makes the lungs less efficient and the heart work harder. A major food toxin to the liver is animal fat including butter.

People who do breathing exercises without attending to the liver may be inadvertently trying to make the lungs do the work of the liver? They can't. But the lungs and liver ARE synergistic. They need each other. You need both to live. Take the breathing tests before and after a liver cleanse and see how they are influenced by the liver cleanse.

Spring is a particularly good time to cleanse - So is any other time except perhaps winter.- Living foods begin to surface from the ground in spring. We replenish our minerals and food enzymes with fresh raw organic fruits and vegetables in solid and fresh juice form. Raw is mostly better but moderate cooking such as stir-frying is better than no fruits and vegetables at all.

This liver cleanse procedure has been in the public domain for many generations. It effectively and painlessly removes stones, gravel, crystals and debris that hinder healing and the ability to detoxify pollutants from the gallbladder and the liver and cleanses the liver bile ducts.

Purpose:

Cleansing the liver of gallstones dramatically improves digestion — the basis of your health. You can expect many or all of your allergies to disappear, with each subsequent cleanse. Each liver cleanse "cures" a different set of allergies, suggesting that the liver is compartmentalized - different parts having different duties. It follows that by getting all the stones out, all allergies will disappear! Well - incredibly, a liver cleanse has eliminated shoulder, upper arm and upper back pain.

Introduction:

One of the top jobs of the liver to make bile, 1 to 1 1/2 quarts in a day! The liver is full of tubes (biliary tubules) that deliver the bile to one large tube, the common bile duct. The gall bladder is attached to the common bile duct and acts as a storage reservoir. Eating fat or protein triggers the gall bladder to squeeze itself empty after about twenty minutes (or after ingesting the liver cleanse solution) and the stored bile finishes its trip down the common bile duct to the small intestine and eventually to the colon (large intestine). Of course the gall bladder does not hold enough bile to neutralize all of the liver cleanse solution you have ingested and the empty gallbladder signals its master, the liver, to dump all available bile forcefully into the common bile duct as well and in this fashion the liver turns itself practically inside out and empties all of its available bile together with stones, gravel and crystals to condition that potent liver cleanse solution. The Epsom salt serves to relax the tubules so that the passage of larger stones is painless and smooth.

For many persons, including children, the biliary ducts (tubing) are choked with gallstones. Some develop allergies or hives but some have no symptoms at all. When the gall bladder is scanned or X-rayed, nothing is seen. Typically, the worst stones are not in the gallbladder but in the liver. Not only that, most are too small and not calcified, a pre-requisite for visibility on X-ray. There are over half a dozen variety of gallstones, most of which have cholesterol crystals in them. They can be black, red, white, green or tan colored. The green ones get their color from being coated with bile. Notice in the picture (of Dr. Hulda Clark's books) how many have imbedded unidentified objects. Are they fluke remains? Notice how many are shaped like corks with longitudinal grooves below the tops. We can visualize the blocked bile ducts from such shapes. Other stones are composites - made from smaller ones - showing that they regrouped in the bile duct some time after the last cleanse.

At the very center of each stone scientists found a clump of bacteria, suggesting a dead bit of parasite might have started the stone forming. Maybe it is the liver's method to encapsulate parasite adults to avoid getting destroyed by such an invader. That's fine for one or two, but how about thousands of such encapsulations?

Eventually the fine self-defense turns into an immense blockage that keeps the liver from detoxifying and eliminating harmful substances such as solvents and parasites. You see, as the stones grow and become more numerous, the backpressure on the liver causes it to make less bile which is of course the transportation medium for the undesirable substances. Imagine the situation if your garden hose had marbles in it. Much less water would flow, which in turn would decrease the ability of the hose to squirt out the marbles. With gallstones and liver stones, much less excess cholesterol leaves the body and cholesterol levels may rise.

Also, gall/liver stones, being porous, can pick up bacteria, cysts, viruses and parasite stages that are passing through the liver. In this way, "nests" of infection are formed, forever supplying the body with fresh irritating bacteria. No stomach infection such as ulcers or intestinal bloating can be cured permanently without removing these stones from the gallbladder and liver.

Preparation:

Cleansing the liver bile ducts is the most powerful procedure you can undertake in order to improve your body's health. A liver cleanse should be done twice a year if possible. Ideally, it should be part of a semi-annual liver/parasite cleanse the sequence of which enhances the overall results.

Phase I (optional): Though some are not sensitive to amalgam fillings, people who are should have dental work first, if possible. Your mouth should be metal free and bacteria free and all cavitations should have been cleaned. A toxic mouth can put a heavy load on the liver, burdening it immediately after cleansing. Eliminate any tooth problem first for best results. If this is not possible then go to the liver cleanse anyway.

Phase II (also optional): Completing a parasite cleanse before cleansing the liver is also highly recommended but not mandatory. You want your kidneys, bladder and urinary tract in top condition so they can efficiently remove any substances incidentally absorbed from the intestines as the bile is being secreted.

About Parasites.

Dr. Hulda Clark maintains that you can't clean a liver with living parasites in it and that you won't get as many stones out, and you may feel quite sick. While this is Dr. Clark's recommendation, it is to me an "ideal" situation. We have seen many stone discharges without the parasite cleanse prior to the liver cleanse.

There are a few good parasite programs. Hulda has one that is tops. Also are Arise and Shine - as a general cleanse or Paragone, Get a stool test from your health professional or http://www.directlabs.com

Phase III (mandatory):

Drink fresh, organic un-pasteurized apple juice for three days preceding the liver cleanse. For these three days, eat frugally (little) if you must and then only small amounts of raw unprocessed fruit and/or vegetable salads, but every day take at least one full quart of high quality unfiltered (you should be able to see the sediments on the bottom of the container) preferable home-made apple juice. The pectin in the apple juice helps to soften and flatten the stones in the gall bladder and liver. This will also help their passage through the bile ducts. This semi-fast also empties the intestines of their food content and makes the collection of stones less problematic. Use a good juicer and make up 20-30 pounds of apples into juice and refrigerate.

If sugar from the juice in relationship to candida is a problem I believe that doing this cleanse is senior to candida worries - for three to four days - as it helps rid the body of parasites. Candida is a parasite as well. Diabetes or severe reactions from this cleanse need special guidance from a professional nutritionist. If you have candida and must take fruit juices then take copious probiotics and Threelac while you cleanse.

LIVER CLEANSE INGREDIENTS:

- Epsom salts 4 tablespoons (not less!!!)
- Olive oil 3/4 of a cup (light olive oil is easier to get down, use only the best cold pressed virgin oil)
- Fresh grapefruit and lemons. Do not use concentrate or store-bought juice. Make your own. Enough to squeeze 1/4 cup of lemon and 1/2 cup of grapefruit juice.

• Ornithine (optional) 4 to 8, to be sure you can sleep. Suitable jar with non-metallic lid. Shake your mixture well and gulp it down 1/2 cup of lemon/grapefruit juice Use a couple of ounces of this juice each time to help get down the Epsom salt solution (four feedings) if desired.

Phase IV - (Procedure):

Choose a day like Saturday for the cleanse so that you can rest the next day.

- Take no medicines, vitamins or other pills that you can do without except probiotics. They could hinder success of the cleanse. Stop any parasite or kidney cleanse the day before.
- Eat a no-fat fruit breakfast and light fat-free lunch such as cooked cereals with fruit but no butter or milk. This allows the bile to build up and develop pressure in the liver. Higher pressure pushes out more stones.

2:00 PM. Do not eat or drink after 2:00 o'clock. If you break this rule you could feel quite ill later. Get your Epsom salts ready. Mix 4 tablespoons in 3 cups of water and pour this into a jar. This makes four servings, 3/4 cup each. Place the jar in the refrigerator to get ice cold (this is for convenience and taste only). If you are familiar with the procedure, take an enema before 4:00 PM with distilled (not chlorinated) warm water to clean out your large intestines of any unwanted fecal matter. The cleaner your intestines are the easier it will be for the stones to be eliminated. Besides, if you want to see just what you will be eliminating it is more appetizing to look only for stones and not be turned off by other smelly stuff.

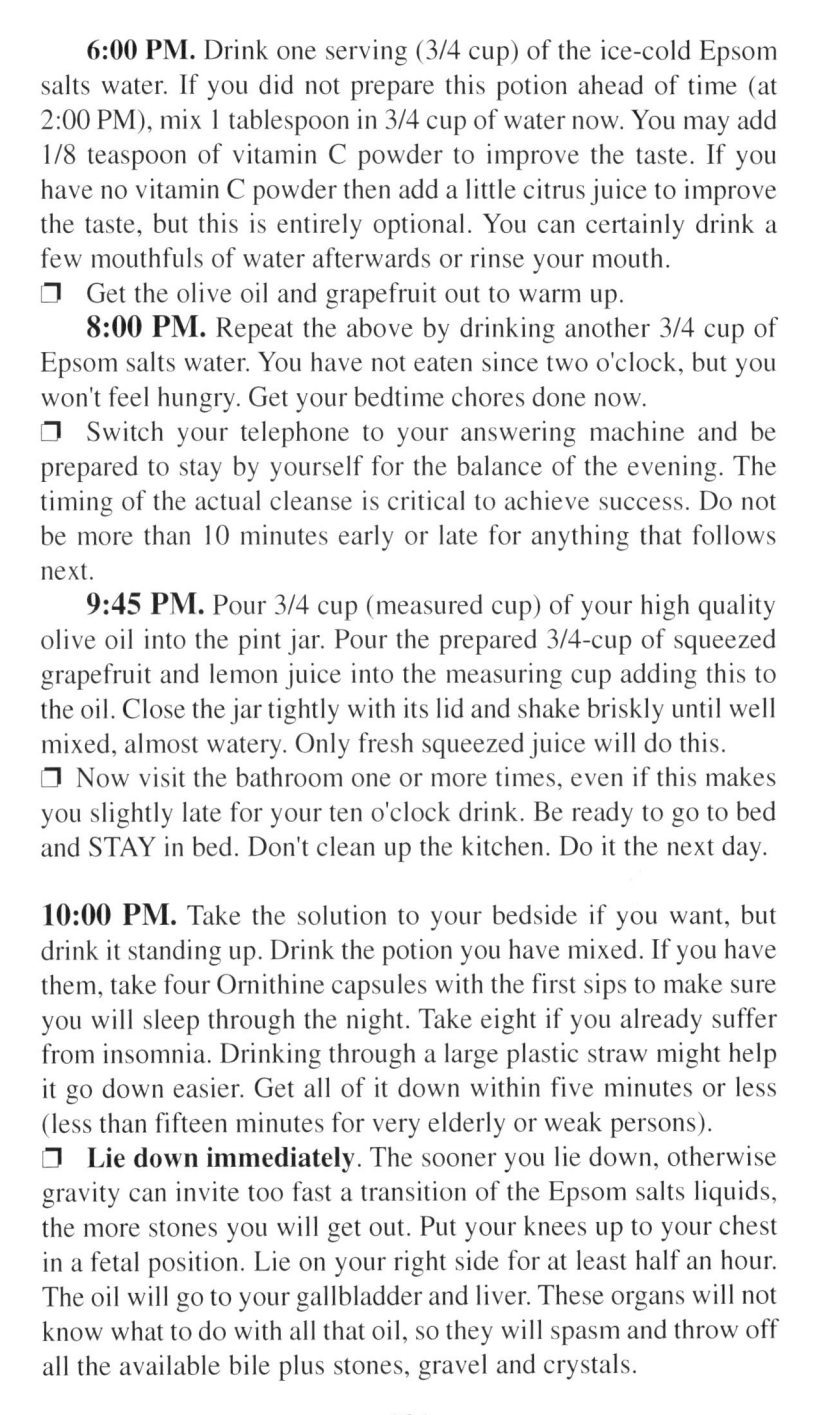

6:00 PM. Drink one serving (3/4 cup) of the ice-cold Epsom salts water. If you did not prepare this potion ahead of time (at 2:00 PM), mix 1 tablespoon in 3/4 cup of water now. You may add 1/8 teaspoon of vitamin C powder to improve the taste. If you have no vitamin C powder then add a little citrus juice to improve the taste, but this is entirely optional. You can certainly drink a few mouthfuls of water afterwards or rinse your mouth.

❐ Get the olive oil and grapefruit out to warm up.

8:00 PM. Repeat the above by drinking another 3/4 cup of Epsom salts water. You have not eaten since two o'clock, but you won't feel hungry. Get your bedtime chores done now.

❐ Switch your telephone to your answering machine and be prepared to stay by yourself for the balance of the evening. The timing of the actual cleanse is critical to achieve success. Do not be more than 10 minutes early or late for anything that follows next.

9:45 PM. Pour 3/4 cup (measured cup) of your high quality olive oil into the pint jar. Pour the prepared 3/4-cup of squeezed grapefruit and lemon juice into the measuring cup adding this to the oil. Close the jar tightly with its lid and shake briskly until well mixed, almost watery. Only fresh squeezed juice will do this.

❐ Now visit the bathroom one or more times, even if this makes you slightly late for your ten o'clock drink. Be ready to go to bed and STAY in bed. Don't clean up the kitchen. Do it the next day.

10:00 PM. Take the solution to your bedside if you want, but drink it standing up. Drink the potion you have mixed. If you have them, take four Ornithine capsules with the first sips to make sure you will sleep through the night. Take eight if you already suffer from insomnia. Drinking through a large plastic straw might help it go down easier. Get all of it down within five minutes or less (less than fifteen minutes for very elderly or weak persons).

❐ **Lie down immediately**. The sooner you lie down, otherwise gravity can invite too fast a transition of the Epsom salts liquids, the more stones you will get out. Put your knees up to your chest in a fetal position. Lie on your right side for at least half an hour. The oil will go to your gallbladder and liver. These organs will not know what to do with all that oil, so they will spasm and throw off all the available bile plus stones, gravel and crystals.

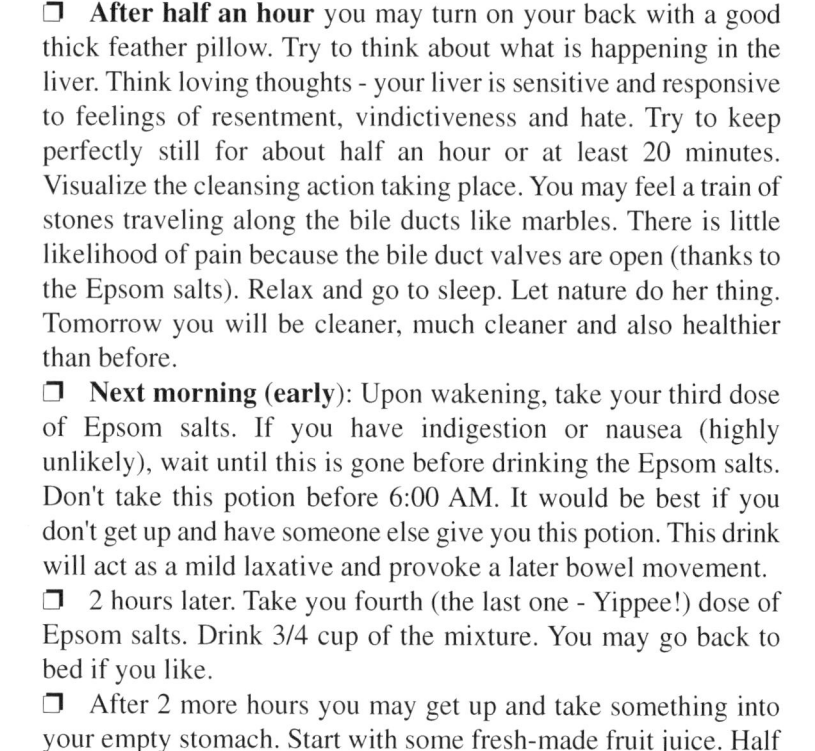

❏ **After half an hour** you may turn on your back with a good thick feather pillow. Try to think about what is happening in the liver. Think loving thoughts - your liver is sensitive and responsive to feelings of resentment, vindictiveness and hate. Try to keep perfectly still for about half an hour or at least 20 minutes. Visualize the cleansing action taking place. You may feel a train of stones traveling along the bile ducts like marbles. There is little likelihood of pain because the bile duct valves are open (thanks to the Epsom salts). Relax and go to sleep. Let nature do her thing. Tomorrow you will be cleaner, much cleaner and also healthier than before.

❏ **Next morning (early)**: Upon wakening, take your third dose of Epsom salts. If you have indigestion or nausea (highly unlikely), wait until this is gone before drinking the Epsom salts. Don't take this potion before 6:00 AM. It would be best if you don't get up and have someone else give you this potion. This drink will act as a mild laxative and provoke a later bowel movement.

❏ 2 hours later. Take you fourth (the last one - Yippee!) dose of Epsom salts. Drink 3/4 cup of the mixture. You may go back to bed if you like.

❏ After 2 more hours you may get up and take something into your empty stomach. Start with some fresh-made fruit juice. Half an hour later, eat some fruit. One hour later you may eat regular food, but keep it light and natural. By supper of the next day (Monday) you should feel fully recovered and ready to slay a dragon.

How well did you do?

Expect diarrhea in the morning of the second day (Sunday). The ideal way to see what you are actually eliminating is to defecate into a white porcelain bowl or large white plastic bucket. The bowl or bucket is used to also see the reddish crystals which collect at the bottom of the bowl (the stones float on top) and those crystals would ordinarily be lost somewhere at the bottomless hole in the toilet and you would have missed them. The alternative is to use the toilet and look into it for the stones with a flashlight. Look for the greenish kind since this is proof that they are genuine gallstones and not food residue.

Only bile from the liver is green. The bowel movement (if there is any) sinks but gall and liver stones float because of the cholesterol inside. Count them roughly, whether tan or green. You may have to eliminate up to 2000 stones before the liver is clean enough to rid you of allergies or bursitis or upper back pain permanently. The first cleanse may rid you of them for a few days but as the stones from the rear of the liver travel forward they might give you the same symptoms again. You may repeat this gallbladder/liver cleanse at two-week intervals until no more stones come out. **Never cleanse when you are ill**.

❐ Sometimes, the bile ducts are full of cholesterol crystals that did not form into round stones. They appear as a "chaff" floating on top of the toilet bowl water. It may be tan colored, harboring millions of tiny white crystals. Cleansing this chaff is just as important as purging stones. We don't know what is the identity of the reddish heavy small crystals that collect at the bottom of the bowl.

How safe is the liver cleanse?

It is very safe. Dr. Clark's opinion is based on over 500 cases, including many persons in their seventies and eighties. None went to the hospital; none even reported pain. However, it can make you feel quite ill for a one or two days afterwards, although in every one of these cases the maintenance parasite program had been neglected. This is why the instructions direct you to ideally complete the parasite and kidney rinse programs first.

Conclusion:

The above procedure contradicts many modern medical viewpoints. Gallstones are thought to be few, not thousands. They don't get linked to pains other than gallbladder attacks. It is easy to understand why this is thought: By the time you have acute pain attacks, some stones are in the gallbladder, are big enough and sufficiently calcified to be seen on X-ray, and they have caused inflammation there.

http://www.curezone.com

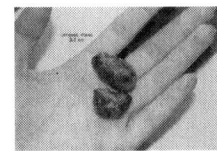

When the gall bladder is removed, the acute pain attack is gone but bursitis and other pains and digestive problems remain and get worse. Stones are not thought to reside in the liver. If the liver is operated upon only the biggest and worst offenders can be removed - yet uncountable stones and gravel and crystals remain in the already clogged liver which has not improved at all.

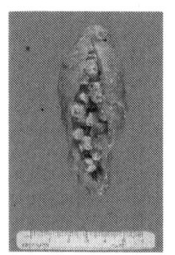

❐ People who have their gallbladder surgically removed still eliminate plenty of green, bile-coated stones with our liver cleanse and anyone who cares to dissect their stones can see that the concentric circles and crystals of cholesterol match textbook pictures of "gallstones" exactly.

http://www.curezone.com

Note:

If you feel waves of pain reaching up to your throat, you probably have a gallstone stuck in a bile duct (clay-colored stool is evidence of bile duct blockage). Epsom salts can relax that bile duct in 20 minutes. Take a tablespoon in 3/4 cup of water but only on an empty stomach or you may feel quite ill. Taking a large dose of valerian herb (6 to 8 capsules four times a day including bedtime) may also buy you a little time by relaxing the duct. If you do get relief, you can be sure it was a spasm of the bile duct system.

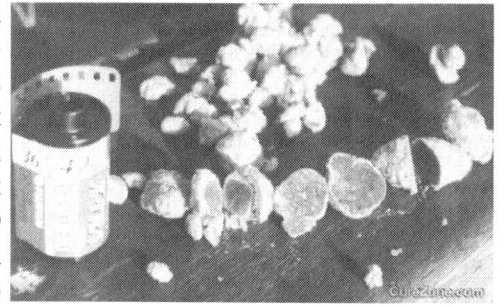

ALL photos on this page are from http://www.curezone.com

The magnesium in the Epsom salts relaxes spasms. It would be best to clean the liver a number of times (at two week intervals unless too ill) to try to dislodge the sticking gallstone. Usually it is recommended to kill parasites and cleanse the kidneys first.

❐ A quick word about parasites: infested humans, pets coupled with international travel, help spread parasites. They are much more predominant than in early non-airplane days. For parasites try both **Oxycleanse** http://www.breathing.com/programs.htm or your local health food store.

To obtain permanent liver health, one should control the intake of high fat foods such as ice cream, potato chips, salad dressings, cheese, butter (excess), cream and exorbitant amounts of milk (more than 1 glass a day, if any). Feelings of resentment, vindictiveness, belligerence and hate are destructive to liver health. Avoid these at all cost!!! Forget the 'bad' others have done to you and forget the 'good' you have done to others. Learn to forgive!

The Cure Zone http://www.curezone.com Large discussion board on a WIDE variety of topics!

CHAPTER 14
Weight Control

The secret to how much you weigh is what you put in your mouth. If you ate nothing (fasting for, instance) for 3 months you would most certainly lose weight — a lot of weight!

2 to 5x T-shirts are a sign of rampant malnutrition. We are the most overfed nation on earth. Many feed their emotions with their fork and spoon.

Self-evaluation of respiratory deterioration was significantly predictive of death from all causes. Kauffmann F, Annesi I, Chwalow J -Epidemiological Research Unit INSERM U 169, Villejuif, France. European Respiratory Journal 1997 Nov; 10(11):2508-2514

In other words there are ways of telling yourself how good your breathing is and what you observe is related to how long you may live due to good or bad breathing. Body weight is one of them.

About 50 percent of your energy goes to digestion when you eat! <u>If you get TIRED when you eat – you're eating too much!</u>

If you wolf down your food, your stomach has to work double or triple time. The Wigmore Institute in Puerto Rico (one of my favorites) dedicates part of their program to proper chewing.

Lacking energy? Drink a quart of water – it's full of oxygen –H_2O -(with 1/8 to 1/4 tsp. sea salt) 1/2 hr. BEFORE eatingÉ <u>**NOT during eating**</u> as <u>**water and other liquids dilute stomach acids**</u>.

Eat SMALL (preferably mostly RAW) meals, chew THOROUGHLY (50 times per bite) and watch your energy levels go UP! And the POUNDS come OFF!

Alkalize your body and the weight just slips away – EASILY!

ELIMINATE sugar, un-pasteurized dairy, chocolate, alcohol, and all grains. Watch your weight go down.

Rather than focusing on *"losing weight,"* a better resolution is to learn to live lean, which will mean some lifestyle changes. The following are my top tips for easy lean living: **Hint**. The secret is largely what you
DO NOT eat. But let's first start here.

Include natural, high-fiber foods and "good" fats in your eating plan, such as the monounsaturated fats and omega-3s that I think are best, such as those in salmon you can get mailed form Vital Choice in Washington.

Make fruits and vegetables a focus–not an afterthought–in your daily menu. 3 pounds or more daily. Substitute Bariani olive oil for butter in your cooking.

Add more fiber to your daily routine. It will keep you feeling satisfied longer, reducing hunger cravings. I use 4 tablespoons of freshly powdered flax seeds daily. The days I do that I experience craving for breads, sweets, and other foods that are not good for me. A meal replacement shake of fresh fruits, spinach, collard greens, celery, and a green powder from Fred Bisci **866 RAW DIET**, http://www.rawfoods.com or E3live http://www.breathing.com/e3live.htm plus plant based protein powder like hemp seed or fermented soy powder or fresh almond milk. Make it so it tastes great or you will not drink it for more than a few days or weeks.

Keep moving. Exercise at least four hours a week. Simply walking and completing light workouts with weights will do wonders for your weight. For more exercise tips see the Secrets of *Optimal Natural Breathing Development* Manual. Add an oxygen concentrator http://www.breathing.com/oxygen-concentrator.htm to you stationary bike, treadmill or cross trainer. Do our daily 6 breathing development exercises from the 176 video/DVD program. Alternate it with the exercises in the manual and/or Get Carolinda Witt's *T5T* book

Drink lots of water. The centers of the brain that interpret hunger and thirst are next to each other. . Most of the time, if you are eating properly, your craving for food and snacks, is your brain telling you — YOU ARE THIRSTY! **Your physical yearning is not so much from hunger, but from dehydration.** More about this in the water section.

Fresh organic foods are best. Avoid non-organic, processed foods, foods containing chemicals, trans fats, most spices and preservatives.

Toss all coffee including decaffeinated and substitute green tea. The nutrients in green tea will help you burn more calories at rest. "Friends don't let friends drink Starbucks" is one of my favorite bumper stickers.

Supplement your metabolism using vitamins, minerals, and nutrients. Nutritional support is crucial to feeling well as your body weight is changing. Some of the best weight management nutrients include green tea, magnesium, and chromium. To make it easy to get all of these nutrients in one place, we prefer one formula. See the supplements section in this writing. It is important to remember that while I think these nutrients are important in achieving weight loss, they're only part of a program that includes eating the right foods, avoiding the bad ones, and exercise.

Set up a support system. The greatest weight loss successes occur when people had friends, family, and counselors constantly offering encouragement and positive reinforcement.

Sleep well. Fatigue causes us to look for cheap imitations of energy like caffeine and sugar. Get our sleep book http://www.bresthing.com/sleep-book.htm

138

Experiment with supervised fasting. http://www.breathing.com/fasting.htm or a local Naturopathic Doctor.

Twice yearly do a complete detoxification program

In *"Raw Family,"* a book written by the entire Boutenko family of four, Victoria, Igor, Sergie and Valya, Sergie's body was cured 100% of "Junior Diabetes" within 4 months time. The family doctor said Sergie was incurable!

All four members of the Boutenko family had a major illness when the family started with their switch from a "normal" (these "normal" people worry me) cooked food diet to their commitment to raw food. All four soon left their diseases behind. In time as their bodies became more alkaline, the mother and son, both very, very overweight, lost most excessive fat and moved from being heavy-footed to light-footed walkers and joggers instead. Victoria lost almost 100 pounds in her first 6 or 7 months as a raw-fooder. A 100% raw food diet is one major way to return back to a natural and permanent life-long alkaline-LIFE base. It can keep weight on though if you include too many sweet and oil dishes.

Learn which foods are alkaline and which are acid. **Keep your daily diet consisting of at least 80% alkaline foods and liquids!** START WITH THEM. This means lots of fruits and veggies, less meat, non unsprouted seeds or nuts, and far less non wild animal protein foods, no alcohol, no coffee or other such acid forming foods and drinks, and certainly no smoking!

For your body get akaline forming products such as **Miracle's Neutralizer, Miracle Soap, Moisturizing Soap, Miracle Gel, and Miracle Skin Moisturizer.** Anyone, even a baby can use 7 drops to a half oz. or more of Neutralizer daily without any adverse health effects.

If you would like to order Miracle 2 products, go to: http://www.global-lightnetwork.com/store/shopaff.asp?affid=364
TOLL FREE order line: **1-888-236-2108**   Use Affiliate ID #364

OBESITY AND BREATHING

Effects of Obesity on Respiratory Resistance (increased force required to breathe and shortness of breath). *Chest* 1993 May,103(5):1470-1476. These findings suggest that in addition to the elastic load, obese subjects have to overcome increased respiratory resistance from the reduction in lung volume related to being overweight. Numerous measurements have shown that the low pO_2art resulting from stressful events or following degeneration of the lung heart system (LHS) in old age can be re-elevated up to high values. Manfred von Ardenne - *Stress* 1981 Vol. 2 Autumn.

Dr. Robert Young's fabulous new book **The pH Miracle for Weight Loss** is due out in July 2005.
Order it here: http://www.innerlightinc.com/vizual

REMEMBER:

"The secret of weight control is what you put in your mouth and how often you chew each bite."

CHAPTER 15
Lung Diseases

Be careful here. Many "diseases" are miss-diagnosed and many others are prescription drug induced. See the **Bantam Pill Book** and this writing for more about the drug aspects. Unless you have had recent surgery to your trunk area or have a hole in your lung, then you had better consult a lung surgeon about that, you can be sure when you have a breathing problem, you will most often want to develop your breathing. The main issues are - better now and precisely just how.

EMPHYSEMA?

I start with this because when you know how to improve the worst cases then the easier ones become just that — easier.

Dr. Robert Nims, M.D., now retired chief of pulmonary medicine at West Haven Veterans Hospital in Connecticut says this about the respiratory clinical study he participated in: *"The standard teaching was that air trapped in the emphysematous lung was trapped and could not be exhaled. For this reason the diaphragm was pushed down to a flat position and the ribs were elevated. Now I told Carl in no uncertain words that he was 'mildly demented' to say that he could effect a rise in the diaphragm and a descent in the ribs, but we got rather spectacular results showing that he did do this."*

Emphysema is fairly simple to slow or stop its progress. This should instill hope for others with varying forms of Chronic Obstructive Pulmonary Disease including pleurisy, pulmonary fibrosis, sarcoidosis and others. Get 2nd and third opinions so that when you improve the diagnostician(s) can not cop out and say you were miss-diagnosed in the first place and never had the illness you thought you had and were taking all the drugs and steroids for.

Some breathing exercises have contained and backed off shortness of breath classified or miss-classified as emphysema. Some breathing exercises have made it worse. That insight carries over into so called healthy people. It tells me that some exercises that work for those that appear to be healthy but are not really healthy "breathing wise" are causing stress harm or inviting illness that is not detected until later in life.

A small number of people with emphysema are born without a lung-protecting enzyme called alpha1-antitrypsin. This makes them more likely to develop emphysema at an earlier age. This may make raw foods critical to optimal health but I am not sure which foods contain the above mentioned enzyme.

SMOKING DAMAGE

The Framingham study proved that **smoking accelerates lung tissue damage by as much as 50%**. It also proved that when smoking ceases, the acceleration stops. But most often by then the lungs have had severe loss of function.

Can this lung function be returned? Even a great deal of it? Yes. Either by developing what you already still have or reactivating what you thought you lost but did not lose. I mentioned this elsewhere but let me say again that I smoked a pack and a half of unfiltered camels a day for 14 years. That was 35 years ago and now at age 64 and 6'2" inches tall the American Thoracic Society says my lung volume is that of a 6'10" 20 year old.

Is it easy? Maybe yes maybe no. Is it worth it? You have to answer that for yourself. How important to you is your breathing and your life span? You need to do simple daily breathing development techniques plus general overall movement type exercises that activate the breathing system in a non-stressful way. You need to cleanse, have a great diet and exercise moderately if you want to achieve optimal results.

Whether you are ill or not the daily breathing regimen will expand the lungs and invite extra energy to do the more active exercises. The gentle but more active exercises will help flush out toxins in the body, including the lymphatic system. Recommended Program http://www.breathing.com/stop-smoking-program.htm

ASTHMA

Asthma, like most things health wise, is what I call multi-factoral. It has several components.

❏ Gather 100 people in a poorly ventilated room with major air pollution and only a few would become wheezing, gasping or "asthmatic".
❏ Gather another 100 group together with poor diet and still only a few would become wheezing, gasping or "asthmatic".
❏ Gather 100 people with emotional problems and only a few would wheeze, gasp or "asthmatic"..
❏ Gather 100 people with poor breathing mechanics and internal coordination and many more will have shortness of breath symptoms than in the food or air group.
❏ Gather 100 with poor breathing mechanics (UDB), poor air, unresolved emotions, and poor diet and you would have most of the group wheezing gasping or "asthmatic".

The underlying cause of asthma is often not air or food, it is the way people are breathing in the first place. It is most often but not always one of the easiest components to improve. Kind of simple really. The mechanical part of asthma is like having a hungry python wrapped tightly around your chest and/or your muscles not responding in a way that allows you to breathe deep, balanced and easy.

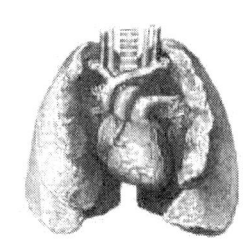

See the lungs (left) and notice how they are mostly in the sides and back and not much in the front — even when you add back the cutaway portion. So it is largely a great waste of time trying to get any breath in the upper chest.

One essential difference between asthma and COPD is that the lungs have been damaged or are plugged up more with COPD. **Asthma is more about breathing in the high chest which has very little lung tissue and causes vaso constriction which closes the airways.** This causes anxiety, caused by trying to breathe improperly. The more a person tries to breathe that way the harder it is to breathe. This is where anxiety turns to grabbing for the inhaler and/or often into panic. Panic attacks are largely breathing pattern (UDB) issues.

Emphysema (you may as well include it in COPD) comes primarily from damaged lung dysfunction as well as high chest or massively uncoordinated, poorly sequenced breathing, compounding and confusing the issue. Nutrition and cleansing is VERY important, as you learned in the digestion and elimination chapter. Emphysema often settles in the lower lobe area but also in the middle or lower middle where the "Speed Bump" is felt. See this article: http://www.breathing.com/articles/breathwave.htm

Stress and asthma are joined at the hip because stress causes the unbalanced breathing patterns (UDB) to be focused upward into the high chest, adding to vaso constriction, causing restrictions in chest muscles, veins, arteries and capillaries.

Stress Places Asthmatic Children in Danger http://www.mercola.com/2004/dec/8/stress_asthma.htm The occurrence of stressful events in a child's life can multiply his or her risk of asthma attacks four-fold.

Makes sense. Inhalers and steroids only muffle the symptom(s). The cause of the factors listed below must be addressed.

According to Dr. Mercola;s article, *"The negative effects of stress can definitely harm a child's mental and physical health. According to a study, stress caused by threatening, upsetting or unsettling life events could quadruple a child's risk of asthma attacks."*

Such stressful events include:
* Moving
* Births/deaths
* Departures
* Illness/hospital visits
* Separations
* Changes in family relationships

During the study, 60 children (ages 6-13) who suffered from asthma for at least three years were analyzed. Throughout the study's 18-month time span, the children were advised to keep a diary and record any acute asthma attacks and their breath strength (peak flow). The children received check-ups every three months and their parents were questioned about potentially stressful events occurring during the corresponding time period. Results of the study showed that the traumatic events were associated with spells of acute asthma.

BRONCHITIS

Bronchitis can be viewed as an advanced form of an aspect of asthma. They often get confused for each other. There is even a name for that called asthmatic bronchitis. COPD is an advanced form of either/both.

Beginning with mechanical function (remember the python), much of the bronchitis approach works well with asthma. The bronchioles need a good cleansing and love a good bug killer. They are to me more critical then the lungs because they are main airway passages and if they are plugged there is no air to the lungs in the first place. So bacteria killers like ones mentioned in the nutrition chapter that keep those airways open are critical to proper lung management as well as emergency applications.

ANTIBIOTICS & BRONCHITIS

Background: Despite the findings in controlled trials that antibiotics provide limited benefit in the treatment of acute bronchitis, physicians frequently prescribe antibiotics for acute bronchitis. The aim of this study was to determine whether certain patient or provider characteristics could predict antibiotic use for acute bronchitis in a system where antibiotic use had already been substantially reduced through quality-improvement efforts.

Methods: A retrospective chart review was performed in an academic family medicine training center that had previously instituted a quality-improvement project to reduce antibiotic prescribing for acute bronchitis. Patients who had acute bronchitis diagnosed during an 18-month period and who had no other secondary diagnosis for respiratory distress or a condition that would justify antibiotics were selected from a computerized-record database and included in the study (n = 135). Charts were reviewed to document patient symptoms, physical findings, provider and patient characteristics, and treatment.

Results-Thirty-five (26%) patients received antibiotics for their acute bronchitis. Adults were more likely to receive antibiotics than children (34% vs. 3%, P < .001). Analysis of 20 different symptoms and physical findings showed that symptoms and signs were poor predictors of antibiotic use. Likewise, no significant differences were found based on prescribing habits of individual providers or provider level of training.

Conclusion: In a setting where antibiotic use for acute bronchitis had been decreased through an ongoing quality-improvement effort, it did not appear that providers selectively used antibiotics for patients with certain symptoms or signs. Other factors, such as no clinical cues, might drive antibiotic prescribing even after clinical variation is suppressed. [J Am Board Fam Pract 13(6):398-402, 2000. © 2000 American Board of Family Practice]

From Mike: I get bronchitis. The last bout I added our Respiratory Enhancer to the water bottle of my oxygen concentrator. I put in 5 drops and breathed it for 10 minutes, no reaction. Added 5 more drops and breathed it for another 10 minutes; much phlegm produced. Added 5 more drops and breathed it for 10 minutes, more phlegmbut not as much as before. Added 5 more drops and breathed it for 10 more minutes. Three day continuous coughing stopped. Started again in 5 hours, did 10 drops in fresh oxygen concentrator water and no more coughing. No guarantees but it sure worked for me.

REGENERATING ALVEOLI with nutrition — instead of drugs

Scientists funded by the National Heart, Lung, and Blood Institute have demonstrated a remarkable regeneration of alveoli, which returned to their normal size and number. In research using rats at the Georgetown University School of Medicine, treatment with retinoic acid, a metabolite of vitamin A, resulted in a non-surgical reversal of damage caused by emphysema for the first time. Not only was the number of alveoli increased in normal rats, but alveoli in rats with emphysema were repaired, and lung elasticity recoil was significantly improved. Though these studies have so far been conducted only in animals, results are very promising, leading a number of physicians to put their emphysema patients on retinoic acid therapy.

This points to why many people live quite well following strict nutritional guidelines, moderate exercise and optimal natural hygiene.

I am confident that this remarkable nutritionally based therapy will be more widely adopted. In fact, the FDA may be approving all-trans-retinoic acid for emphysema therapy. All-trans-retinoic acid must be prescribed by a physician.

UPPER RESPIRATORY TRACK

The "acid rain" of the body is what lodges in the sinuses. The mouth, throat, nasal passages plus mostly the sinuses collect "debris" as well. Most people don't realize that the sinuses are huge and go way back into the head.

When the sinus cavities get full of bacteria, the bacteria travels down the throat, past the larynx into the bronchioles and lungs. This causes or worsens speech problems, bronchitis and lung congestion.

I recently worked on a man's breathing mechanics who started coughing and spitting up mucous for 45 minutes. I encouraged him to continue to do so. I had opened the lungs and they then allowed the backpressure to subside. This backpressure of inflammation in the lung area was causing the sinuses to stay plugged. His voice got clear and strong for the first time in 8 years. His sinuses cleared up as well.

Poor Digestion and Elimination cause similar "debris" problems.

See separate chapters about them.

ELIMINATE any mucous producing food such as dairy, bread (anything with white flour), red meat, grains and chocolate. More about this in the nutrition section.

I have asked a world-class aroma therapist to create for me an essential oil formula called **Respiratory Enhancer**. It comes in two forms. One for rubbing on to the chest and the other for inhaling via an oxygen concentrator. It's really good for the lungs. (More about this at http://www.breathing.com/oxygen-concentrator.htm) It's really good for the lungs but not to replace any traditional medical approaches although the aroma therapists The oils in this formula are all good bacteria killers.

When people who want to focus a lot of attention to their respiratory system come to my office, I have them combine the far-infared sauna, O2 generator, Respiratory Enhancer and alternate with low impact aerobic exercise. (A rebounder is good for this!).

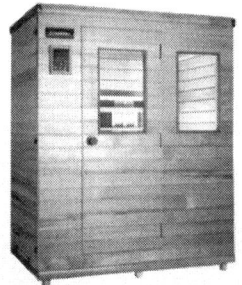

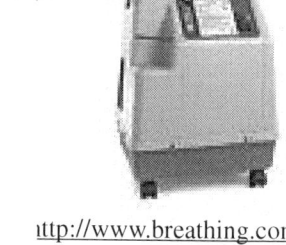

http://www.breathing.com/sauna.htm

http://www.breathing.com/oxygen-concentrator.htm.

http://www.breathing.com/rebounder.htm

148

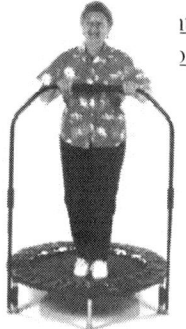

CHAPTER 16
Lung Toxins Hiding In Over 300 Prescription Drugs?

Remember — if you had a negative side effect and you did not take a prescription drug they would call it a disease. Side effects are diseases, pure and simple.

300 Prescribed Medicines Can Damage the Lungs
http://www.breathing.com/articles/pneumotox.htm

This warning was issued at the first World Congress on Lung Health and Respiratory Diseases in Florence, Italy, where 15,000 specialists from 84 countries gathered during the week of Sept. 3-9, 2000. Their official statement was clear, "There are hundreds of medicines routinely prescribed for a variety of disorders, including high blood pressure, allergies, rheumatism, certain cancers or even common non-respiratory inflammations, that can cause all kinds of lung diseases." These diseases are classified as accidents that are induced in a patient by a physician's prescribed treatment. These diseases may develop in a very short time. They are mostly unpredictable and some are irreversible, leaving lifelong damage.

Judging by the 4,200 bibliographical references collected by a team at the University Medical Center in Dijon, France, **there are no less than 50 different lung diseases and syndromes (ranging from simple coughs and breathlessness to pleurisies and even acute respiratory failures) that seem to be either caused or aggravated by medicines.** Also, each year there are no less than 20 to 30 new therapeutic substances being added to the list of suspect products.

The Dijon, France, team goes on to say, *"The information provided with the packaging hardly ever warns patients that the medicine could potentially cause a lung disorder and, there are very few doctors who give this matter due consideration when they prescribe a treatment."*

According to the specialists attending the World Congress in Florence, - with an early withdrawal of the medicine, about 70% of cases would increase the patient's chances of avoiding a damaging disease or condition.

Medicinal herbs and some supplements have even been blamed for serious lung problems. There are also some therapeutic treatments that appear on this list, such as blood transfusion, laparoscopy, acupuncture, the insertion of catheters and various body punctures.

Professor Camus of the University Medical Center explained at the World Congress in Florence, *"These accidents could largely be avoided, or at least reduced, but only if certain conditions are satisfied.*

First*, the practitioner who has been consulted (whatever his specialty) must be aware of what has happened.*

Second*, the patient has to consult as soon as he notices the slightest abnormal or lasting pulmonary symptom.*

Third*, and last, the patient must immediately stop taking the suspect product, which is absolutely essential if lasting harm is to be kept to a minimum."*

A Dijon, France, team has put together a unique, regularly updated Internet site which makes all this information available to patients and practitioners free of charge. Every month this website is visited by 6,000 to 7,000 visitors, half of which are from the United States.

Below is just the A list of A-Z of drugs that may injure the respiratory system.
Go here for the link to the rest. http://www.breathing.com/articles/pneumotox.htm
Abacavir
 Abciximab
Acebutolol

Acetaminophen (= paracetamol)
Acetylcysteine
Acetylsalicylic acid
Acrylate
Acyclovir
Adenosine and derivatives
Adrenaline (= epinephrine)
Albumin
Allopurinol
Almitrine
Aminoglutethimide
Aminoglycosid antibiotics
Aminorex
Amiodarone
Amitriptyline
Amphotericin B
Ampicillin
Amrinone
Anagrelide
Angiotensin converters enzyme inhibitors
Antazoline
Anti-inflammatory drugs (non steroidal)
Anti-lymphocyte (thymocyte) globulin
Anticoagulants (oral) (= Warfarin)
Antidepressants (also see specific drugs)
Aprotinin
Atenolol
Aurothiopropanosulfonate
Azapropazone
Azathioprine
Azithromycin

CHAPTER 17
Oxygen Therapies
Otto Warburg

Since Otto Warburg received the Nobel Prize in 1931 for proving cancer can not survive in a high concentration of oxygen, science has been investigating oxygen and its healing powers... only not very much or very well.

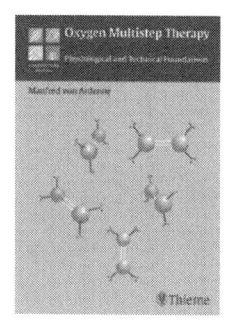

Warburg's prize student Manfred von Ardenne was an electron physicist who in addition to his interest in astronomy, developed quite a good reputation for cancer research . He worked for decades creating what he called **Oxygen Multi-step Therapy,** which focused on oxygen's relationship in to most major categories of illness. When your blood oxygen goes way down, you get sick, die or at best shorten your life span.

This book is a masterful compilation of clinical insights and variations on breathing assessments, cofactors and some techniques of breathing development. In this book Dr. von Ardenne addressed some 150 respiratory and blood gas aspects including elements of what we might call respiratory psychophysiology.

Germs, fungi and bacteria are anaerobic as well. von Ardenne was also inspired by Karl Lohmann who discovered adenosine triphosphate, ATP, which many believe to be the human body's main energy currency.

Some studies addressed in the book include:
- Dependence of O2 uptake at rest.
- The O2 deficiency pulse reaction as a warning sign of a life threatening crisis, and the lasting remedying of the crisis.
- Procedures that influence and measure increases and decreases in arterial and venous O2 blood levels.
- The necessary physical exercise to attain a training effect. (less

than you might believe)
- Increases in brain circulation during physical strain.
- Rate of blood flow in the circulation of the organs.
- Various examples in changes of O2 uptake.
- Heart minute volume and blood flow of the organs decisive for O2 transport.
- Relation of ATP concentrations in rat brains as a function of the oxygen partial pressure of the inspired air.
- He graphed much of his research.
- Other cofactors that influence lung volume are airways hyper-responsiveness, atopy, childhood respiratory infections, air pollution, posture, subluxation of the spine, exercise, deep and superficial fascia, nutrition, occupational hazards, abuse and trauma, attitude, and age, height, weight and sex.

Because of this I created a program combining a used oxygen concentrator with a Far Infrared Sauna and Stationary Bicycle or Cross Trainer or Treadmill. You can learn more about this at www.breathing.com/oxygen-concentrator.htm

Ed McCabe

The next person to address oxygen in a huge way is investigative reporter Ed McCabe. His *Oxygen Therapie*s published in 1984 sold over 250,000 copies and set the stage for his *Flood Your Body With Oxygen* published in 2003. No other person comes even close to gathering and clarifying oxygen's power as a healing force. I believe Ed deserves a Pulitzer, Nobel Prize or at least national recognition for this work!!

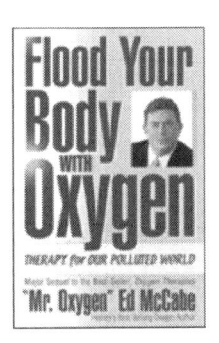

Hyperbaric Oxygen Chamber pioneer

Another prize for courage under fire should go to Robert Hartsoe of http://www.miraclemountain.org His hyperbaric oxygen chamber treatments are one-tenth the cost of most hospital treatments!

Remember that the best way to get oxygen is to breathe optimally.
The next best way is with water and living foods.

CHAPTER 18
TESTIMONIALS
...from satisfied private session clients and self help customers

"I am a 69 year old MD Ear Nose Throat specialist who developed adult onset asthma and "non reversible airway disease". I could not get any real help except inhalers. I came across Breathing.Com from Stephen Sinatra's Newsletter. I ordered #176 DVD and have tremendous improvement. I do not get winded doing simple tasks. My wife and I do Tai Chi at 5 AM everyday. I also agree with Mike regarding the raw food diet and drinking a lot of water. I believe that chronic dehydration is another key to aging and in my case lung disease. I took the breathing school this year and am involved in helping people help themselves. That proper breathing is the first step in wellness seems so logical but is most frequently overlooked. Keep up the good work Mike!" — **Randall Langston, M.D.**

"Most people tend to breathe in the upper chest, stimulating the sympathetic (flight or fight) nervous system. This inefficient breathing begins at birth and increases with conditioning, civilized life's non-stop emotional upheaval, polluted cities and increased stress. Using Optimal Breathing techniques, we bring our breath down and learn to return to the parasympathetic (slowing down, restorative) nervous system, helping us to stay balanced on all levels. Through learning how to breathe in the whole body we go beyond the mind into the realms of spirit, thus cultivating divine inspiration." — **Philip Madeley,** Tree of Life Educational Manager, http://www.treeoflife.nu

SPASMODIC DYSPHONIA

"I am a 46 year old Speech and Language Pathologist who ironically acquired a severe voice dysfunction following a severe throat infection. As a professional, I had learned about this "rare, incurable neurological disease" called Spasmodic Dysphonia, which was resistant to treatment and devastated the lives of those afflicted. Fortunately, I knew there were professionals that did offer a cure (without the frequently used injections of Botox which offer temporary relief) and so I began my quest for restoring my voice. I first consulted Dr. Morton Cooper in Los Angeles. Dr. Cooper is also known as the Voice Doctor and has authored many articles and books. He has for years attested to the fact that many people, when they learn to use their voices in an optimum manner, can overcome the disabling effects of Spasmodic Dysphonia and he has many testimonials to his credit.

I worked with Dr. Cooper for several days and he gave me hope and set me on the right track with his simple exercises. I then consulted with Robert Grider of Minnesota Voice and Speech Clinic. I trusted Bob because he was a friend as well as a fellow SLP and he added some exercises to my regime, primarily use of a quiet, confidential voice and some other techniques to decrease the strain, struggle and hoarseness inherent in SD. Both Dr. Cooper and Bob had some very simple breathing exercises they prescribed, but I expressed concern to both that I felt that my breathing was "stuck" and shallow, and try as I might to "belly-breathe", I felt I needed something more. I took up Yoga and the deep breathing which did seem to help, but I continued my search.

*A search on the internet led me to Mike White's **Optimal Breathing Program** website. I emailed Mike right away, and he was easily accessible and encouraging. I took an on-line quiz and found that I had what Mike calls Unbalanced Deep Breathing. I ordered Mike's video and manual and realized that what I needed to develop was full, optimal breathing and that there were simple exercises to trigger the deep breathing reflex.*

I met with Mike personally and did a three-hour private session during which he addressed my voice difficulties and performed some more in-depth work. I highly recommend Mike's program, and since I believe that most if not all people with SD do not use their breath optimally, I feel it is of significant benefit with this population. Seven months after the onset of my SD, I have regained a fairly functional voice, and am presently working on increasing my loudness and further improving voice quality. Typically a direct voice rehabilitation program for SD can take 6-12 months or longer, but I definitely do not consider it an "incurable" disorder. Like the voice, so many of our body systems are linked to our breathing and Mike's manual is quite comprehensive in both explaining the anatomy and physiology of breathing. Along with his video, Mike provides easy ways to achieve better breathing, and outlines multiple applications and benefits."

— **Connie Pike, MA, CCC-SLP** Tampa, Florida

Comments from Optimal Breathing School core faculty member.

DONNA GROSS

"My background includes thirty years of experience in Holistic Care with licensing in Respiratory Care and Personal Training. I have worked ventilators in critical care and I was the therapeutic specialist in a Pulmonary Rehabilitation Program. I ran a senior's Wellness Program teaching Yoga, Tai Chi and Chi Gung. I trained under and worked as a therapist for the founding President of the Holistic Medical Association. I also have worked for other doctors using Naturopathic and Ayurvedic therapies.

All this experience has taught me a lot about health as well as disease. I know the power and limitations of medical treatment in the field of pulmonary health. Most of the effective treatments are useful in acute or emergency situations. They have limited success in long-term health management. For example, most of the breath testing done on pulmonary patients has to do with forcing an inhalation or exhalation to record air flow. Forced breathing causes increased tension in the lung tissue. This is not a healthy practice in a patient already suffering from high levels of tension in the lungs.

This same principle holds true with many of the medications given patients. A Bronchodilator can save a life by forcing open swollen airways, but it cannot improve anyone's overall state of health if used regularly. Eventually the patient fails to respond to the chronically used medications, and the possibility of tissue damage from these medicines increases as they are used year after year, decade after decade.

We try to teach clients to find the underlying causes of their breathing problem. Then they can work to improve their immune system and develop improved life style habits. The idea is to wean off the medicines eventually. It takes someone with an open mind and a brave spirit to travel this path toward healing. This is the road less traveled, and it is unique to each individual. It seems to me to be the path of beauty and well worth the effort, if one is truly intending to heal."

Success Stories Results, Testimonials.
Taken from the http://www.breathing.com/results.htm page

Optimal Breathing incorporates the best of all breathing development techniques and exercises. The people we work with come from a cross section of almost every job, race, religion, or lifestyle on earth. Optimal breathing is generic to ALL humanity. The results-success stories-testimonials on the following 3 pages will give you more insight into the broad range of breathing development applications.

TESTIMONIALS OVERVIEW

A **champion swimmer** wanted to improve her ease of breathing and recovery times for multiple general race days and championship tri-athlete events. An **opera singer** was losing her high notes and sought psychotherapy but eventually just learned to breathe better and her high notes returned. A **classical singer** was losing her mid range and regained it with optimal breathing techniques. An **emphysema victim** learned that breathing was not what he thought is was, for over 50 years. It had become a permanent misunderstanding even to the point of doing it improperly when shown the proper way. Sixteen sessions were needed to change this person's breathing. An **asthmatic** was retrained to breathe easier and the symptoms disappeared. **Stuttering** and **spasmodic dysphonia** can reduce or disappear when one learns to breathe optimally. **A shy young lady** learned to breathe better. Her shyness lessened and "I met a man and got married". Some eliminated their **sleep problems**, **hypertension**, **type "A" responses**, wimpy ways of being. Some **increased their energy** many fold, told off their suppressive boss, told the truth to their spouse, opened up to loving themselves, and set boundaries where needed. Some healed from illness or near death. There are thousands of stories like this below.

Singing

I was recently singing to Phantom of the Opera and some Barbara Streisand and then some other music. What I noticed is that the high notes which didn't used to be all that clear, are amazingly strong and clear – all the time. I can easily and powerfully reach a high "A" which before could easily be a struggle. And it's a clear sound, not screeching to reach it. This is so amazing! I love it. This is the voice I have always wanted. And in ONE session as well.   – Pamela Tablak, Soloist and Choir Director Recommended Program http://www.breathing.com/consulting.htm

Asthma, Emphysema, Anxiety, Insomnia

"Breath is the essence of life. When we expire, we lose life. When we are inspired, we gain life. The art of optimal breathing can provide a great contribution to the art of optimal living.

Michael Grant White has been studying the science and art of breathing for two decades and is a masterful teacher. His training materials, workshops, and personal coaching sessions provide insights which can transform lives.

I was amazed to learn how much benefit can be gained in chronic diseases such as asthma, angina, emphysema, anxiety, and insomnia thru the application of Optimal Breathing strategies.

I'm glad to be able to endorse Michael Grant White's highly evolved program of Optimal Breathing. However, as with any program that requires application, the benefits you gain are

generally proportional to consistency with which you practice these principles. If you are ready to fulfill your life potential, I recommend you begin by fulfilling your breathing potential."
— **James Biddle M.D.** Diplomat, American Board of Internal Medicine Diplomat.
 Also practices chelation therapy and preventive medicine. http://www.integrative-med.com

I am a changed Person
"I would like to thank you very much. I am a changed person. I watched the video and did the first exercise it was just what I needed. I sleep better, look better, and think better, all because of the video and exercise #1. I will try the others later, You are really doing some wonderful work, is there an exercise for weight loss? I need to read more of the manual. God bless you for the help, its just wonderful. Thanks again!" — Wanda Chafin Recommended program for weight loss: http://www.breathing.com/weight-loss-program.htm

Adrenal exhaustion, anxiety
"I am a 58 years young woman, high school teacher, and have spent much of my life off and on going through periods of adrenal exhaustion (of which I really had no name for up until a few years ago) and wondering why I couldn't catch my breath, actually have to crawl up stairs sometimes, waking up at night breathless etc.

This all would come to pass when I was going through some kind of loss or what I perceived as a loss, or just any old time especially during times of a great deal of change. Interestingly enough when I was not going through those times, I have amazing energy, accomplish a great deal and rarely get tired. It became clear to me about 15 years ago that losing my mother at 3 years of age and not being told until I was 5 where she went, and simply living in hell with my father in one of those abusive long term dysfunctional stories (tragic but boring) put me in so much fear that I learned to hold my breath and do all of the stuff that goes along with the flight or fight syndrome.

Long story short approximately 10 years ago described these symptoms to my doctor, adrenal surges, not being about to catch my breath, waking up at night many times gasping for air and feeling like I am suffocating was put on Zoloft or Paxil off and on for about 10 years. I would tell the doctors, that I didn't feel depressed and really had no idea why these physical symptoms would happen to me and be so debilitating, but they just treat symptoms with meds. People would tell me, well just take a deep breath. OK I'll do that I would say but I could n not seem to get a handle on being able to get a real breath when I'm suffering t h is panic and anxiety.

One fine day last October it finally dawned on me, I do not know really HOW to breathe! With all of the Yoga, meditation, bodywork, no one has been able to really teach me "HOW TO BREATHE". So I got on the WWW and said help!!! Punched in "breathing" and, 'Walla' came "breathing.com" and Michael. Got Michael's tapes in his Breathing kit http://www.breathing.com/breathingkit.htm

Breathing Exercise Tape #1 http://www.breathing.com/exercise1.htm was such a shock for me, what I mean is I had no idea there was a reflex action at the bottom of the exhale breath that actually "breathed your body". The shallow breathing that I was in the habit of doing had never allowed the development of that reflex action. So naturally I'm waking up at night breath holding, panic stricken and clueless why this is happening.

My body has been oxygen-starved and getting worse as I get older. EVEN THOUGH ALL OF THE CHILDHOOD ISSUES ARE WORKED OUT, GONE, DONE WITH, the old breathing habits had remained, I was not aware of something better.

Breathing Exercise #2 http://www.breathing.com/exercise2.htm was even more fantastic! The exercise uses what you have learned in tape #1 and gives you the tremendous tools and power over the physical disablement of being oxygen starved and emotionally stressed.

Very soon after starting the tapes, I visited Michael for 6 days in North Carolina to get private instruction. I can only tell you all that it was the best thing I could have ever done for myself. I am now of course still practicing proper breathing (50 years of bad habits), off meds, and have not awaked at night even once since starting the tapes and getting private instruction from

Michael.

Again Michael, thank you a million times over for actually dedicating your life to helping people understand the importance of the breath and actually in detail showing how to really practice it.

— Phyllis Ross Recommended program. http://www.breathing.com/energy.htm Level 3.

COPD

*"Thank you for sending the "**Secrets of Optimal Natural Breathing**" to me so promptly. I did get it in plenty of time to take it to Cape Cod with me. There I simply read it several times without trying to do any exercises or assessments. In the past few days I have been trying to work with the exercises. I have also worked with the tape once. I intend to continue all this because already I have had some significant help. I do plan to come up for some individual work in the next few months. I am quite taken back by your work. I recently finished a pulmonary rehab program at Vanderbilt University; and this morning when I walked (hobbled for a few blocks) I thought: "Well everything I did in that program was a kind of forcing; and now for the first time, I am glimpsing what it means to take a real breath." When I got home my oxygen saturation jumped up to 99% for the first time.*

Thanks a lot! I have a long way to go. In addition to my COPD I am now struggling to recover from a back injury. I will continue with your basic exercises for a while and let you know when I might make a trip."

— Phyllis P. Recommended Program http://www.breathing.com/energy.htm Level 4

Emphysema

"I read all of your information and pretended I was on the beach watching the ocean just like you said. When I received your study I tried each exercise. I visualized my lungs as hard and crusty and the only way to improve was breaths from my knees to the top of my head with long exhales and letting the in breath come in by itself.

With a little improvement each day I am attempting to stomach breathe while walking. The more I convince myself that the cause of my improvement is deep breathing -----the more I extend the time I deep breathe each day. I am walking up to one mile daily now. "Many thanks, Mike."   D.L. Emphysema. Victim

From Mike: This gives us good insight but is not necessarily universally appropriate.
Recommended Program   http://www.breathing.com/energy.htm Level 4

Orthopedic Specialist
"I thoroughly enjoyed my session with you. I was delighted by the degree of insight and sophistication that you bring to "breathing". I am now opening up and breathing in a much more relaxed I look forward to another session to go a step further. I will also be recommending your approach to my patients." — Dr. Richard Gracer, Orthopedic Medicine. Walnut Creek, California.
Recommended Program http://www.breathing.com/school.htm

Chest Pains, Shortness of Breath, High Blood Pressure
"I have tried emailing this testimonial sometime in May but somehow it never got through. Since then my daughters have been urging me to send in my testimonial because of how much your breathing exercises have helped me "cure" my chest pains, shortness of breath and lower my blood pressure. So I am sending it in now hoping this does get through to you.

I need to thank God for leading me to your website when I began experiencing mild to severe chest pains every night. I had gone through a full bottle of 30 nitroglycerine tablets within two weeks. My chest pains always occurred at night when I am going to bed, so much so, that I was afraid to go to bed.

I need to explain something, Mike. Because of my past two open heart surgeries and heart problems, I am quite knowledgeable about the symptoms of a possible heart attack when you experience chest pains. In my case, I had just gone

through an ultra sonic and a treadmill test in February. During the treadmill test, at the final stage, I complained to the attending nurse that she had to stop the treadmill because I was experiencing severe chest pains and was out of breath. She insisted I continue because the test is almost over and I needed to go on just for another minute or so. Somehow I got through the run and nearly fainted, heaving and breathing rapidly.

Two weeks later when I returned to my cardiologist for the results of my test, the cardiologist stated that I had over 75% blockage on my right carotid artery and 50% blockage on my left carotid artery. He immediately recommended an angiogram to determine the actual extent of the blockage. After consulting with my wife, I decided to forego the angiogram and in fact vowed that I would not go through that invasive examination again. Right after that was when I started to experience my chest pains. However, as I mentioned to my wife, the chest pains that I was experiencing could not be heart related but instead, I suspected it may be initiating from my lungs.

After my treadmill test, I also started to cough out some mucous. Its color was pure white and not yellow or black so I felt that I may have a latent lung problem. After all, I am over 73 tears old. Besides during my chest pains, I did not experience any of the usual symptoms of a pending heart attack. I felt like I couldn't breathe and the center of my chest hurt badly. The pain vanished after I slipped a nitro tablet under my tongue. My blood pressure was not low at the time but it wasn't high either. Of course I was frightened. I would get chest pains for two or three nights, then none on the next night, and then it started again. About that time, I read an article in our local newspaper about breathing.

I went on the internet and I can't tell you how or why I selected your web site. I spent all day reading the information on your site especially the testimonials. I ordered your Optimal Breathing package and received the tapes in early April.

Now, let me tell you what happened. I started out on the middle of my living room floor, arranging some couch pillows on a towel on the floor. Didn't take me long to adjust myself on the floor and started with the **Better Breathing Exercise #2** recorded *audio.* As God is my witness, by the time I was into the second half of the tape and into the exhale and inhale on a single bong strike, my right leg from my thigh to my feet felt like ice. I continued my breathing exercises and had my wife cover my legs with a blanket. I went through the entire exercise which took me nearly an hour that very first time.

Mike, that night I did not have any chest pain. I did the same exercise twice the next day, once in the morning and then again before going to bed.

The second night, my chest pain returned, but this time instead of taking a nitro tablet, I went into the living room and sat on the edge of my couch and in the dark, started to breath slowly. The chest pain slowly subsided and after a few minutes it was gone and I was able to go to bed. From that day on I have had no chest pains and have not taken a nitro tablet. This all happened in April after I started with your breathing exercises.

Today, I do breathing almost the entire day, mostly subconsciously be causing the breathing exercises is part of my daily routine. There is a lot more I can tell you about my health as a result of the breathing exercises I learned from you.

My daughter who lives in Hawaii has just visited you in North Carolina and I am grateful for the teaching and help you have given her. I have told my youngest daughter about the (Better Breathing Exercise 2) and she too will be doing the healing breathing exercises herself. In closing here is my email address, bobby7778@hotmail.com for anyone who is fortunate enough to find your website, they can contact me and I would be happy to tell them how wonderful breathing the right way can do for them!"* Aloha, — **Bruno Yim**   Recommended Program http://www.breathing.com/energy.htm Level 3. Level 4 if you need alternative health supplements

Breathing, Trauma & Personal Power
by Alan Paul

"I was a long-term severally abused child, physically and emotionally. I am steadfastly determined to improve my sense of wholeness, to strengthen my self-esteem and self-love and spiritual connection with others. As a result of this commitment, I have spent much of the last 30 years looking for help with my breathing, which has always (since adolescence) felt tense and shallow and "locked up" and eventually led to me having to give up my chosen profession.

Over the years, I've tried every type of healing modality I could think of that might impact the experience of never being able to get a satisfying breath. I've tried medical doctors, chiropractic, and various psychotherapies including Psychoanalytic, Gestalt, Short-Term Psychodynamic, and others. I've tried body-oriented therapies including Reichian, Alexander Technique, Rebirthing, , Rosen Work, Biofeedback, Massage Therapy, Bioenergetics, Core Energetics, Primal, Reiki, Cranio-Sacral, etc.. I also studied Yoga and Tai Chi. For many of these modalities I tried more than one practitioner of that style. I also committed extensive periods of time to a number of these practitioners, many of whom I studied with for periods of 1 to 3 years, in hope of getting some help.

While some of these teachers and therapists were very smart and dedicated people who were able to help me move forward in one way or another, no one was able to help me find relief from my core complaint my inability to breathe satisfactorily.

I recently discovered the website of breathing.com and opened a dialogue with Michael Grant White, the director of the site. Eventually, I decided to travel to North Carolina for a week, to work intensively with Mike.

Mike started by showing me how some simple adjustments to my posture could give me more space to breathe. He then, using very specific rib/chest/shoulder/neck accessory breathing muscle release techniques went on to show me how to get the ribs and diaphragm moving so that the breath could expand into the increased space he had found for me in my posture. Some of the beliefs that I had held about what a coordinated breathing feels like, had to be corrected. Finally, there was a wonderful moment with Mike when everything "clicked" for me, and I was able to sing loudly and happily with no pain or straining, for the first time I can remember since early childhood. Mike was able to get me back to the same state again, and I eventually returned home with a set of exercises and "homework" to do to help continue the development. I was quite satisfied and happy with my lessons with Mike.

But the biggest changes became apparent when I returned home. Suddenly, conversations with associates had a different character, the movement of my ribs seemed huge compared to before I traveled to North Carolina. A close associate has commented that I seem noticeably more relaxed. My dreams are much more vivid (some pleasant, some not so pleasant). A low-grade depression seems to have lifted, and I suddenly find myself easily working long hours whereas that was difficult for months before my trip.

I've also noticed an odd and unexpected difference in my diet after years of complacency, I've begun eating salads every day and generally eating less overall. Food is still very enjoyable, but it seems less like entertainment and comfort to me, and more like...well...food. Somehow, breathing a little deeper and easier has, without any conscious effort to do so, made me more realistic and less emotionally clouded about diet.

Another thing that changed immediately after returning home, is my exercise routines. I generally swim every day and do a good bit of flexibility work every day. But after studying with Mike, I'm beginning to feel that there really is only one form of exercise breathing development. Everything else (swimming, stretching, weight-training, tai chi, running, you name it) is just a variation of breathing development.

For example, when I swim now, I'm very conscious of moving my limbs and ribs in such a way that the breath deepens with every stroke, so that the breath is more expansive and elastic when I get out of the pool than when I got in. This is quite different than the way I used to swim. I swam a lot harder than I swim now, and there was a general sense of triumph and temporary relaxation in that, but the relaxation didn't extend to my breath, which was tight and shallow when I was finished. Mike has assured me that I'll swim even stronger than before, if I'm careful to slowly increase the cardio demand such that the breathing apparatus remains relaxed. I always thought that the more cardio fitness, the better, as long as one doesn't have a heart attack. But I've learned that you can do quite a bit of subtle damage to the enjoyment of your life (and even your long-term health) by placing athletic demands on your body that are out of synch with your breathing abilities. So breathing comes first for me now, particularly since Mike's given me some tools with which to increase my breath.

I've noticed the same thing with my stretch routines. I no longer believe that there's such a thing as an "ankle stretch." Sure, I do the same ankle routines as before, but the way I do them is completely different. So there's no ankle stretches. Just "breath stretches" extended out to the ankles.

Mike also talked to me repeatedly about the ergonomics of my life in my easy chair, my work chair, and my car seat. When Mike discussed these things, I listened and thought he made some good points worth considering. But since I've returned home, I'm beginning to feel that he was talking about something really important_. I can see how slouching at my desk for a couple of hours leaves me with less breath, and that then induces a feeling of low self-esteem and depression. I guess I never noticed before because I didn't feel that I had all that much breath to protect. Now, with my breath deeper, I'm beginning to think seriously about how to improve my ergonomics (Mike gave me a number of good and inexpensive suggestions.)

Just now, as I sat and wrote this, I realized that I am indeed slouching and locking up my breath. I need to replace this desk chair with a more breathing-friendly chair (not a specialty item, just an inexpensive but different chair design than I'm currently using), in accordance with the suggestions that Mike gave me. So I got up and did about 10 minutes of my breathing exercises. Now, sitting back down to work, it's easier to work, the words are flowing with less effort, my self-esteem is higher, I feel more confident, life seems less like a burden. It's subtle, but tangible. No, it's not magic, my life isn't suddenly euphoric. But it's easier, less work, more filled with hope and promise, than it was 10 minutes ago. It makes me wonder how many of my internal conflicts and frustrations are nothing more than the effects of poor breathing habits.

Some people tell me to let go of the past, grieve the losses, forgive those who hurt you, move on toward life. They mean well by encouraging me to fly, but they assume that I have the wings with which to fly. How can I grieve the past and move on, if my breathing is locked up so that I can't fully laugh, cry, or sing?

Mike has helped me see some of the possibilities for correcting my breathing pattern, and the results of that have been simple and immediate. It feels good to breathe better. And it's very reassuring to know that there are specific exercises I can do for my breath, that will help me to let go of the past and create the future." — AP. Recommended program. http://www.breathing.com/energy.htm Level 3. Level 4 if you need supplements.

MEDITATION
Greetings from London, England.
"I have been practicing TM since October of last year. I have also been practicing your Breathing Exercise #1 for the past few weeks since ordering the tape. I enjoy TM but find it's effects variable and occasionally quite negative (although this was pointed out as being natural by the excellent tutor).

years and in just a few weeks of assiduously practicing this one exercise I have received more benefit than in twenty years of practicing all manner of other breathing techniques. Now here's the really good bit. I decided I would try using the "Waking Breath", - Breathing Exercise #1 - whilst doing my TM even though in basic TM practice there is no conscious breath control (the mantra itself is supposed to encourage shallow almost imperceptible breathing).

The result is a totally positive quality of experience both in the meditation session and afterwards. I can't speak for other TM practitioners but the moral seems to be that whatever practice you are engaged in get your breathing right first and it will help and support everything else. It really is the place to start.

I can't thank you enough. (And yes, I am now going through the manual.".

Recommended Product   http://www.breathing.com/meditation-program.htm

M.I.T Trained Biochemist

"Of all the essential nutrients needed by the human, oxygen is the one we must have on a moment-to-moment basis; we can't live without it even for a few minutes. yet, this is the one nutrient most people don't associate with deficiency problems. Nothing could be further from the truth.. One problem is that oxygen concentrations in and around major cities have been measured as much as 30% below normal. That means that each breath brings in less oxygen. As if this weren't bad enough, most people have developed poor breathing habits, thus further restricting oxygen intake.

The resulting oxygen deficiency is having a negative effect on our health and our overall performance. Oxygen deprivation can be associated with all kinds of chronic diseases, including cancer. Michael White is an extraordinary breathing coach who teaches people new patterns of breathing, helping them to bring in more oxygen. These techniques help to improve health, stamina and even voice quality." – **Raymond Francis,** Director, Beyond Health Corporation http://www.beyondhealth.com **From Mike.** Raymond has been quite successful with AIDS victims.

Raw-Living Foods Chef

"I highly recommend the work of Michael Grant White. It has touched my life on a very profound level. Excellent breathing is absolutely essential to everything in our lives. It provides energy, assists digestion, improves>brain efficiency and assists in providing optimal body functioning. Breathing for me though is much more. Breathing correctly has allowed me to tap into the magical side of life... the spirit within!

Through learning how to breathe in the whole body we can go beyond the mind and our animalistic thinking. Most of us breathe in the chest area stimulating the sympathetic (Flight or Fight) nervous system. This incorrect breathing began at birth with our conditioning, civilized life's non-stop emotional upheaval, polluted cites and increased stress without the release.

By learning how to breathe we can bring our breath down and learn to stay in the parasympathetic (slowing down, restorative) nervous system for most of the time. In times of crisis we can use optimal breathing development and exercises to bring it back there.

The practice of Mike's exercises allows the natural reflexive breathing to be rehabilitated. Basically we are retraining our body to breathe naturally, so these are not just short-term exercises, they are designed to recondition and reorganize the way we breathe.

One of the my favorite exercises was not a specific breath exercise, but a Qi Gong exercise. This simple exercise, taught in his Secrets of Optimal Breathing manual, of standing still in relaxed posture has revolutionized my own posture and thus increased my breathing capacity. The Better Breathing Exercise #2 (aka Tibetan Caffeine), http://www.breathingl.com/exercise2.htm , singing exercises and shhh breath in the video http://www.breathing.com/video-strap.htm *(#176 Video/DVD)* have also opened up my breath and lungs like never before.

Two years later I still practice the techniques and exercises because I get results form them!! While working with Mike in 2000 I was introduced to the techniques which really allows an opening and expanding of lung capacity, Mike has a video that you can use at home for this. http://www.breathing.com/video-strap.htm

The changes for me were very subtle, yet like any true natural health practice, accumulative over time. And I have not even practiced them daily!! So don't despair if you don't get immediate results thought many do, just persevere and gradually your breathing will open on a whole new level.

Excellent breathing in conjunction with living foods, yoga and meditation, provides you with the tools that may enable you to find your peace... whatever life throws at you." Philip Madeley   http://www.sattvic-life.com   http://www.freshupnorth.com

Click here for a few words from leading California physician
Dr. Len Saputo   http://www.breathing.com/len-saputo.htm

Chiropractor

"Mike White is truly a master of the breath. As a long time martial artist, chiropractor and singer I thought I had a handle on breathing. What I had in fact was created non-optimal breathing patterns by over emphasizing the abdominal aspect of the breath. This was depriving me of the fullest expansion possible. Mike's due diligence and keen powers of observation helped me open up. As I breathe easier I am letting go of patterns of effort in my life. The breath is truly a living metaphor. Thank you, Mike!". — **David Miller, D.C.**   Recommended Product. http://www.breathing.com/breathingkit.htm

Psychologist Gay Hendricks

"If you've never seen Mike's powerful work, you're in for a real transformational treat. You'll see why he's simply called The Breathing Coach."

Migraines, Chest Pains, Vitality and Emotions.

"Just wanted to tell you how much I enjoy your newsletter. My sister ------ was fortunate to have had the opportunity to meet with you in early June. She mentioned what a kind person you are. She lives in Hawaii, I in Nevada, but we talk with each other several times a week and she has continued working with her breathing. On her way back from North Carolina, she stopped in Nevada to join us in celebrating my daughter's high school graduation, and shared with us what she has learned.

I have had terrible migraines for several years now and just this week, I tried some of your techniques for breathing (properly!) and lo and behold, they first subsided and then eventually disappeared. How wonderful it was to rid myself of this. I will continue these techniques whenever I feel the need.

In closing, please keep me informed if you plan on visiting Las Vegas. My father who also lives in Las Vegas, uses your tapes, etc. as faithfully as my sister and I know he would love to join me in going to any seminars/classes that you may present. He was experiencing chest pains (angina?) periodically and since he started his **Optimal Breathing** *program, he has not touched his nitroglycerine. It is amazing given his history of* *heart disease. He also feels more vital. The greatest reward is that even emotionally, he has opened himself up to us all. I thank you, Mike, as there are many more things that have happened to our family since meeting you."* —**D. M.**

 Recommended program http://www.breathing.com/energy.htm. Level 3. Level 4 if you want supplements.

APPENDIX

RECOMMENDED WEBSITES

1. **BREATHING DEVELOPMENT**
http://www.breathing.com
http://www.authentic-breathing.com
http://www.breathmastery.com
http://www.oxygenysis.org

2. **FASTING & CLEANSING**
http://www.shirleys-wellness-cafe.com/
Shirley's Wellness Cafe
http://www.totalhealthsecrets.com
http://www.tanglewoodwellnesscenter.com
Tanglewood Wellness Center

3. **CLEAN AIR & THE IMPORTANCE OF SUNSHINE • PURE WATER • CLEAN ENVIRONMENT**

4. **BENEFITS OF ORGANIC LIVE FOODS & (WHOLE FOOD) SUPPLEMENTS**
Veteran Raw Foodists
http://www.healself.org   Dr Bernarr- over 50 years
http://www.thegardendiet.com **Storm- over 30 years; Jinjee – 11years**
http://www.superbeing.com   Roger Haeske -over 15 years
http://www.youthing101.com   Viktoras Kulvinskas -over 40 years

Some really GOOD websites for raw foods & recipes:
http://thephmiracle.us
http://www.eatraw.com
http://www.raw-food.com
http://www.rawfoodsupport.com

http://www.relfe.com/recipes.html
http://www.vegetarian-diet.info
http://www.rawfoodfocus.com
http://www.rawfood.com
http://www.living-foods.com
http://www.youthing101.com
http://www.livingnutrition.com
http://www.TheRawWorld.com
http://www.RawFoodsNews.com
http://www.rawfoodfocus.com
http://www.breathing.com
http://www.newveg.av.org
http://www.bestjuicers.com
http://rawbuddy.com
http://www.gogreen.org/
http://raw.tribalglobe.com
http://www.raw.org
http://www.fresh-network.com/
http://www.doctorgraham.cc/
http://www.hacres.com/
http://www.rawguru.com/
http://www.livrite.com/raw.htm
http://www.buildfreedom.com/rawmain.htm
http://www.SuperbeingDiet.com
http://www.vegetarianusa.com
http://www.gardenofhealth.com
http://www.breathing.com
http://www.rawlife.com
http://www.livingfoodsinstitute.com
http://www.lovingfoods.com
http://www.thelivingcentre.com
http://www.visionsofjoy.org
http://www.livefoodsunchild.com
http://www.rawfoodwiki.org
http://www.thegardendiet.com
http://www.sproutrawfood.org
http://www.durianpalace.com/durian-evolution.htm
http://www.thaivegetarianrecipes.com

http://www.celestialrawgoddess.com/
http://www.thebestfoodever.com (coming soon!)
http://www.shazzie.com

Here's where you can find courses on a raw food lifestyle:
http://www.transformationinst.com/
http://www.healthfullivingintl.com/
http://www.tanglewoodwellnesscenter.com
http://www.foodnsport.com

RECOMMENDED BOOKS

1. **WHY SHOULD YOU DEVELOP YOUR BREATHING?**
   The Way You Breathe Can Make You Sick or Make You Well. http://www.breathing.com/theway.htm
   Building Healthy Lungs, Naturally

http://www.breathing.com/bhln.htm
   The Secrets of Optimal Breathing manual
   http://www.breathing.com/secrets.htm
   S.L.E.E.P. — *The Stress Level Elimination Energy Plan*

http://www.breathing.com/sleep-program.htm

2. **FASTING & CLEANSING**
   Toxemia Explained by J.H. Tilden, M.D.
   The Miracle of Fasting by Paul Bragg, N.D., Ph.D.

3. **Clean Air & the Importance of Sunshine • Pure Water • Clean Environment**
   http://www.breathing.com/clean-air.htm
   http://www.breathing.com/articles/canary.htm
   http://www.watercure.com   http://www.nafhim.org
   http://www.ewg.org   http://www.sungazing.com
   Do a web search on Heliotherapy (benefits of sunshine)

4. PERSONAL GROWTH
http://www.breathing.com/bradshaw.htm

5. BENEFITS OF ORGANIC LIVE FOODS & (WHOLE FOOD) SUPPLEMENTS
- *The Sunfood Diet Success System* by David Wolfe
- *Delights of theGarden*
- *Vibrant Living* by Sally Pansing Kravich
- *The Uncook Book* by Elizabeth Baker
- *Raw*
- *Milk Recipes from Nuts& Seeds* by Edith Edwards
- *Vibrant Living* by Sally Pansing Kravich
- *Sweet Temptations* by Frances Kendall
- *Lover's Diet* by Viktoras & Youkta Kalvinskas
- *Not Milks by RobertCohen*
- *Soups Alive!* by Eleanor Rosenast
- *Dining in the Raw* by Rita Romano & Nancy Jolly
- *Hooked on Raw* by Rhio
- *12 Steps to Raw: Breaking The Cooked Foods Addiction* by Victoria Boutenko
- *The Raw Secrets by Frederic Patenaude*
- *The Raw Life* by Paul Nison
- *Living in the Raw* by Rose Lee Calabro;
- *Sunfood Cuisine* by Frederic Patenaude
- *Living Cuisine* by Renee Loux Underkoffler
- *Rainbow Green Live-Food Cuisine* by Gabriel Cousens
- *Sunfood Cuisine* by Frederic Patenaude
- *Living Cuisine* by Renee Loux Underkoffler
- *The High Energy Diet Recipe Guide* by Douglas Graham, Ph.D.
- *Sproutman's Kitchen Garden Cookbook* by Steve Meyerowitz (the Sproutman).

Go to http://www.breathing.com/bibliography.htm for books and links to books on breathing you are looking for.

Gabriel Cousens new book, *Rainbow Cuisine*, talks about different body types on the raw food diet according to his Ayurveda theory and practice (Pitta , Khafa , Vata etc...). This book explains which foods to eat . Cousins also talks about slow and fast oxidizers . This is a wonderful book with research , info , recipes from his center in Arizona. A cerebral book for those who really like a lot of information.   Perhaps your answers lie in these pages .

RAW FOOD & HEALTHY LIFESTYLE COURSES TO TAKE
http://www.transformationinst.com/
http://www.healthfullivingintl.com/
http://www.tanglewoodwellnesscenter.com
http://www.foodnsport.com

KING BIO HOMEOPTHIC PRODUCTS
http://www.breathing.com/programs.htm   (look under homeopathics)
Addicta Plex (promotes nutritive function of brain & nervous system)
Allergy/Hay Fever Reliever
Asthma Freee (Helps relieve shortness of breath, wheezing & tight chest, and mucous congestion)
Lungs & Bronchial Relief
Male Strengthener (helps tone & strengthen male system)
Smoke Control (relieves craving for tobacco, irritability & breathing problems)
Snore Control (fast relief of excessive snoring)

TID PRODUCTS
we order a lot and can probably give you quantity discounts. www.tidhealth.com
http://www.breathing.com/programs.htm
(look under Nutrition & Diet, Cleansing, & Protecting Respiration)

Coral CalMag (coral calcium, magnesium, Vitamin D powder)
Cordyceps PS (Dong Chong Xia Cao)
Emergen-C (Vitamin C & energized minerals)
Inuflora (for discomfort associated with antibiotics)
Oregacillin (respiratory health support)
OxyCleanse (oxygenated colon cleanser)
ProEFA (Omega 3 oils)
ProFlora (Nutritional support for optimal digestion)
ThyMune (supports thymus function)
Vinpocetine (Support for mild memory problems & enhances circulation)

TASTY RAW RECIPES too many to list here!
Here's a few key links to check. These will lead you to others with even MORE recipes!
http://www.living-foods.com
http://www.livingnutrition.com
http://www.rawfood.com
http://www.discountjuicers.com
http://www.rawin10minutes.com
http://www.breathing.com/rawsoups.htm

Optimal Breathing School Core Faculty
http://www.breathing.com/school/faculty.htm

Your improvements on the **Optimal Vitality Goals©** list are best achieved through our Breathing Development Self-Help Programs found at: **http://www.breathing.com/programs.htm** or through personal trainings with an **Optimal Breathing Development Specialist** (find an OBDS in your area at this webpage: **http://www.breathing.com/school/refer.htm**

OPTIMAL BREATHING® SCHOOL
http://www.breathing.com/school.htm

Here's a partial list of modalities that will benefit greatly from attending our school.
Join us and then help us train your colleagues!

Acupressure	Butoh
Acupuncture	Canadian Deep Muscle
Alexander Technique	Chi gung (Qigong)
Applied Kinesiology	Chi Nei Tsang
Aromatherapy	Chiropractors
Ahashiatsu	Colonic Educators
Ashtanga Yoga	Dance Teachers
Aston Patterning	Cranio-Sacral
Barbara Brennan Healing Science	Dance Teachers
Bonnie Prudden Myotherapy	Deep Muscle
Bowen Bodywork	Energy Field Work
Brain Gym	Feldenkrais Method

Feng Shui
 Hatha Yoga
Hellerwork
Holotropic breathworkers
Hypnotherapists
Infant massage
Iyengar Yoga
Jin Shin Jyutsu
Jivamukti Yoga
Jois Yoga
Kinesiology
Kripalu Yoga
Kundalini Yoga
Lymph Drainage
Martial arts. Hard and soft styles
Massage therapists & bodyworkers
Medical Doctors
Movement Therapists
Myofascial Release
Neuromuscular
Nurses
Nursing Assistants
Occupational Therapist
Osteopaths
Pain Relief
Personal Trainers
Physical therapists
Psychotherapists
Polarity Therapy
Power Yoga
Prenatal Massage
Psychiatrists
Psychotherapists
Qigong
Radiance breathworkers
Radix
Raja Yoga
Rebirthing
Reichian therapistsReiki
Reflexology
Respiratory Therapists
Rolfing
Shiatsu
Sivananda Yoga
Speech language pathologists
Stress Relief
Swedish
Tai Ch
Tantra
TCM - Traditional Chinese MedicineTherapeutic Touch
Three in One
Touch for Health
Transformational breathworkers
Trauma Erase
Trigger Point
Tutoring
Voice and singing teachers
Watsu
Yoga in general
Zero Balancing

http://www.breathing.com/school/main.htm

The Optimal Breathing School[a]

LEADING EDGE
TOUCH & NON TOUCH METHODS
<u>Learn how + teach others</u>
Rapidly Develop Natural Mechanical Breathing Function

866-694-6425
(866-MyInhale)

mw@breathing.com

http://www.breathing.com/school/main.htm

Accelerating Healthy Breathing & Speech Development

CEUs* for
Massage Therapists

become an expert in a field few health professionals clearly understand

Mike White's classes address these breathing development problems:

* CEU Progams for other modalities are being applied for.

- **Weak voice** & unable to project
- **Respiratory illnesses** (i.e. bronchitis, asthma, emphysema
- **Symptomatic problems** (i.e. coughing, chronic fatigue, high blood pressure)
- **Mechanical problems** (i.e. cramps in back or neck, hyperventilation, tightness across chest)
- **Emotional symptoms** (i.e. anxiety, depression, shallow breathing)
- **And everything else** that better breathing can influence or control

You will learn to facilitate significant improvement in your own, as well as most client's, breathing - including asthma, COPD, pulmonary fibrosis, and help improve speaking and singing.

Other benefits can include: improved energy, pain reduction, easing pregnancy and birthing, improved sleep, sports performance, stress management, weight loss, stopping smoking, voice strengthening

Optimal Breathing Maximizes
Health & Well Being
Sports Performance
Life Extension
Helps reduce or eliminate need for medication!

Health Professionals
Will gain:
Unique Skills • Better Breathing
Grateful Clients • Additional Income
Increased Client Base • Increased Referrals

My four levels of training address significant aspects of most breathing development problems.

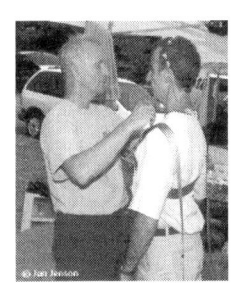

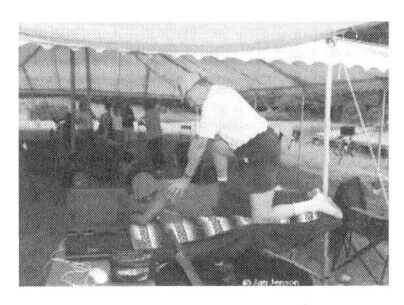

safe * fast * easy * painless

There are many people who have detected breathing problems, such as asthma, COPD, bronchitis — which are easy to spot — but often not easy to improve.

It's the undetected breathing problems that cause the most destruction to a person's health and longevity. These problems act like termites or dry rot because they undermine our vitality and sense of self and allow us to get or stay sick from many other illnesses that use up our oxygen and overtax our nervous, endocrine, digestion, elimination and immune systems.

Take our FREE breathing tests:
http://www.breathing.com/tests.htm

When is the next Optimal Breathing School[a] scheduled?

http://www.breathing.com/calendar.htm

Optimal Breathing®
http://www.breathing.com • 828-456-5689

Our **Optimal Breathing® Development System**[a] utilizes a few breathing exercises, but we found that "exercises" mean different things to different people. Overall "exercise" is a potpourri of good, mediocre, bad, confusing and outright dangerously unhealthy practices for properly developing your breathing. We carefully choose what breathing exercises we DO employ, based on physical function, form and the health, peak performance, self expression, emotional balance and life extension goals of our students and clients.

Manual & Books

191 - **The Secrets of Optimal Breathing**
180 page manual. ISBN #188317-48-1 • **$29** + S&H

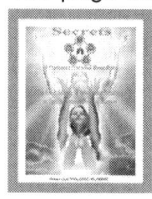

25 years of research related to poor breathing; anatomy; fundamental & accelerated breathing development; exercises -special situations –175 breathing based holistic health programs, (i.e. asthma, bronchitis, shortness of breath); clinical studies; appendix; testimonials

192 - **Building Healthy Lungs, Naturally**
Book. ISBN #188317-50-3 • **$15.95** + S&H

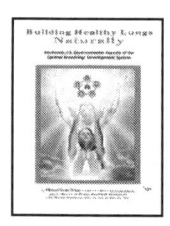

96 page book: Biochemical & Environmental Aspects of the Optimal Breathing® Development System: Cleansing & Fasting; Clean Air, Water & Environment; Organic Live Nutrition & Supplements; Digestion & Elimination; Detox A-Z; Prayer & Meditation; Ergonomics; Exercises; Oxygen Therapies. Over 40,000 breathing tests show that poor breathing is associated with almost ALL health challenges! **How good is your breathing?**

193 - **The Way You Breathe Can Make You Sick! It Can Also Make You Well!**
Book. ISBN #188317-06-6 • **$13.95** + S&H

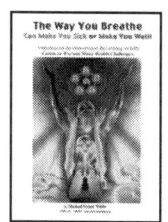

46 page primer exposes breathing problems that begin before pregnancy; air, water, food, exercises, emotions, stress, toxins & trauma affect breathing; myths & cautions; many common breathing problems discussed + LOTS of testimonials!

http://www.breathing.com/theway.htm

194 - **SLEEP Stress Level Elimination Energy Plan**
Book. ISBN #188317-09-0 • **$595** + S&H

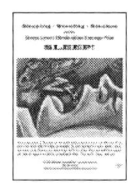

Techniques, exercises, ergonomics, nutrition. Comes with our new S.L.E.E.P. book ($595 value)
http://www.breathing.com/sleep-ebook.htm

DVDs & Videos

176 - **The Art & Science of Optimal Breathing**
DVD or Video - ISBN #188317-41-4 • **$49** pkg + S&H

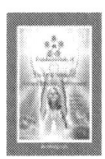

Developing Healthy Balanced Breathing, About diaphragm, exercises, better sleep & relaxation, pain reduction, reduce medication, ease pregnancy, energy increase, stop smoking, weight loss, sports performance, singing & speaking, tests + Begin HERE.

169 - **Optimal Breathing School**[a]
DVD or video. ISBN #188317-42-2 • **$20** + S&H

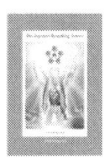

For traditional or alternative health professionals, or those aspiring... you MUST learn optimal breathing development. Advanced training levels being added: personal trainers, singers & speakers, specific modality requirements, Qigong masters and more!

CDs & Cassettes

120 - **Better Breathing Exercise #1**
CD or cassette. ISBN #188317-44-9 • **$15** + S&H

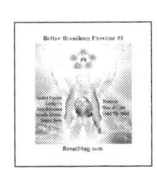

Deep relaxation and deep letting go; learn to rest more easily and deeply; better access your healing state; become more flexible in your thoughts and actions; handling change in a calmer fashion.

130 - **Better Breathing Exercise #2**
CD or cassette. ISBN #188317-43-0 • **$27** + S&H

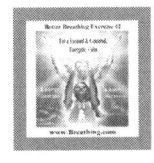

Creating natural energy PLUS focus; energetic calm; more life force energy to increase oxygen, nourish brain, enhance cellular function; jump-start metabolism; speed weight loss & recovery from stress & fatigue; boost sexual energy; be more alert yet non-combative.

140 - **Breathing Self Esteem**
CD or cassette. ISBN #188317-46-5 • **$15** + S&H

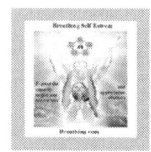

Increased self understanding, opening to the state of flow, alignment between inner and outer expression, comfort with personal expression; acting on authentic self; less perfectionism.

150 - **The Watching Breath**
180 page manual. ISBN #188317-32-5 • **$15** + S&H

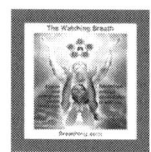

4000-year old meditation - strengthens concentration & deeper awareness; integrating body, breath and mind; better focused thinking; relaxed concentration; calm awareness; opening to a state of slow; being in present time.

170 - **Breath of Life & Vitality**
CD or cassette. ISBN #188317-33-3 • **$15** + S&H

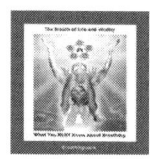

Is there a right way to breathe? Breathing poorly reduces quality of life & life span. Why is deep breathing so misleading to people? Why use inhalers? How to know if you are breathing well? Drug free way to reduce asthma attacks. Importance of nutrition for optimal breathing.

173 - **Raw & Living Foods Festival Seminar**
CD or cassette. ISBN #188317-49-X • **$15** + S&H

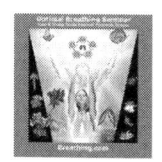

Portland, OR- 2001 Festival. Mike delivers a one hour breathing seminar on CD (no cassettes). Fun and very informative. Anatomy, science, why learn to breathe better. Working on a member of the audience.

195 - **The Way You Breathe Can Make You Sick... or Make You Well!** CD or cassette. ISBN #188317-10-4 • **$15** + S&H   Not available yet

Booklets / eBooks

299 - **Grain Damage**
Booklet   ISBN #1-893831-05-1 • **$7** + S&H

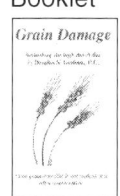

by Dr. Douglas Graham.
Rethinking the high starch diet.
Retail ONLY.

171 - **Optimal Digestion**
Booklet. • **FREE w/orders**

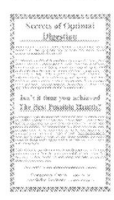

40 page booklet (included in 191 manual or separate) Contains many programs. http://www.breathing.com/programs.htm.

E3Live Super Booster Food
Booklet. • **FREE w/orders**

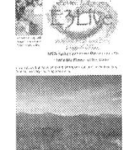

FREE information and bonus gift with first order!
http://www.breathing.com/e3live.htm

Forty-nine Tips
Booklet. • **$5** + S&H (or included with 250 orders)

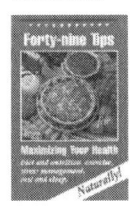

49 great tips on diet and nutrition, exercise, stress management and rest. Start living the healthful life of your dreams today! From the editors of **Health Science** ® magazine - health & dietary principles available nowhere else.

187

More CDs & Cassettes

181 - Prevention & Intention
CD or cassette. ISBN #188317-28-7 • **$15** + S&H

Deep relaxation and deep letting go; learn to rest more easily and deeply; better access your healing state; become more flexible in your thoughts and actions; handling change in a calmer fashion.

130 - Rip Roaring Health
CD or cassette. ISBN #188317-36-8 • **$15** + S&H

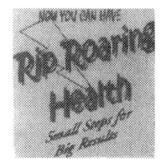

Creating natural energy PLUS focus; energetic calm; more life force energy to increase oxygen, nourish brain, enhance cellular function; jump-start metabolism; speed weight loss & recovery from stress & fatigue; boost sexual energy; be more alert yet non-combative.

160 - Peace Within
CD or cassette. ISBN #188317-30-9 • **$15** + S&H

Opening to the state of flow; peace of mind; sense of well being; improved creativity; decrease anxiety, tension and aggressiveness.

179 - SLEEP Stress Level Elimination Energy Plan
CD only. ISBN #188317-09-0 • **$15** + **$5.95** book + S&H

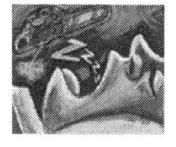

Techniques, exercises, ergonomics, nutrition. Comes with our new S.L.E.E.P. book ($595)
http://www.breathing.com/sleep-ebook.htm

Use our comprehensive way of evaluating your breathing:
FREE BREATHING TESTS: http://www.breathing.com/tests.htm

Wholesale orders — **10 minimum** of any
60% cost of retail price
plus 7% for quantity shipping in USA.
Call about international shipping rates.
CREDIT CARDS Accepted:
VISA • MasterCard » American Express • Discover

http://www.breathing.com/programs.htm
USA Toll Free: 1-866-694-6425
International 828-456-5689
Fax 828-454-5475
P.O. Box 1551 • Waynesville, NC 28786

Unit Prices
#176 DVD & Video - $49
#169 OB School - DVD $15
CDs - $15 • Cassettes - $12
Manual $29 • BHLN $15.95 • The Way $13.95
Sleep $5.95

Qty	Product	Unit $	Total $
___	191 Secrets Manual	$29	___
___	192 BHLN Book	$15.95	___
___	193 TWYB Book	$13.95	___
___	194 SLEEP Book	1	___
___	176 Art OB DVD ___ Video ___	$5.95	___
___	169 OB Sch DVD ___ Video ___	$49 pkg	___
___	120 BBE#1 CD __ Cass __	$15	___
___	130 BBE#2 CD __ Cass __	$15	___
___	140 Self Est. CD__ Cass__	$27	___
___	150 Watch Br. CD __ Cass __	$15	___
___	170 Br. of Life CD __ Cass __	$15	___
___	173 Raw Seminar CD __ Cass __	$15	___
___	195 OB CD __ Cass __	$15	___
	CIRCLE ITEMS THIS PAGE	$15	

Made in the USA
San Bernardino, CA
26 December 2016